# A USMLE STEP 1 REVIEW

# Anatomy

## 10th Edition

W Crane

KUCC

Biology

*A USMLE STEP 1 REVIEW*

# Anatomy

## *10th Edition*

# 700

## *Questions & Answers*

### Jack L. Wilson

*Professor of Anatomy and Neurobiology*
*College of Medicine*
*The University of Tennessee, Memphis*
*The Health Science Center*
*Memphis, Tennessee*

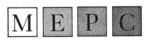

Medical Examination
Publishing Company

APPLETON & LANGE
Norwalk, Connecticut

Notice: The author and the publisher of this volume have taken care to make certain that the doses of drugs and schedules of treatment are correct and compatible with the standards generally accepted at the time of publication. Nevertheless, as new information becomes available, changes in treatment and in the use of drugs become necessary. The reader is advised to carefully consult the instruction and information material included in the package insert of each drug or therapeutic agent before administration. This advice is especially important when using new or infrequently used drugs. The publisher disclaims any liability, loss, injury, or damage incurred as a consequence, directly or indirectly, or the use and application of any of the contents of the volume.

ISBN 0-8385-6218-3

90000

ISBN: 0-8385-6218-3
ISSN: 1079-4093

9 780838 562185

Acquisitions Editor: Jamie Mount Kircher
Production Services: Rainbow Graphics, Inc.
Designer: Mary Skudlarek

PRINTED IN THE UNITED STATES OF AMERICA

# Contents

# Preface

A critical need of medical, dental, and allied health students is to be able to efficiently review and self-evaluate their scientific knowledge of the anatomical sciences and its application to the clinical sciences. The tenth edition of *Medical Examination Review: Anatomy* has been designed with this goal in mind and focuses on examining the student's basic knowledge of the anatomical sciences with emphasis on clinical relevancy and the development of problem-solving skills. The extensive new series of case studies, which have been added to the gross anatomy and neuroanatomy sections, will help the student synthesize and integrate information in solving clinical problems. New illustrations show important anatomical information.

The question format and subject areas used in this book are based on the current USMLE Step 1 examination. The questions are organized into categories to provide a representative sampling of the material covered in each course and will help define areas of strength and of weakness where more attention is needed. For your convenience, answers with commentary and references follow each section of questions. Specific references to widely used textbooks allow you to return to an authoritative source for further study if the brief explanations are not sufficient. The questions and answers, taken together, emphasize problem-solving and application of underlying principles, as well as retention of factual knowledge. I hope that these questions will be a beneficial complement to your studies.

Jack L. Wilson
The University of Tennessee, Memphis

# A USMLE STEP 1 REVIEW

# Anatomy
## 10th Edition

# 1

# Gross Anatomy

## THE HEAD AND NECK

DIRECTIONS (Questions 1–37): Each of the questions or incomplete statements below is followed by five suggested answers or completions. Select the **one** that is best in each case.

1. In which of the following bones are the foramina rotundum, ovale, and spinosum located?
   A. frontal
   B. ethmoid
   C. maxillary
   D. temporal
   E. sphenoid

2. Metastatic carcinoma of the tongue would be expected to spread via the lymphatic vessels directly into the
   A. palatine nodes
   B. deep cervical nodes
   C. gingival nodes
   D. submandibular nodes
   E. parotid nodes

1

3. The artery that enters the cranial cavity through the foramen spinosum is a direct branch of the
   A. external carotid artery
   B. facial artery
   C. lingual artery
   D. maxillary artery
   E. internal carotid artery

4. The primary action of the muscle that originates primarily from the medial aspect of the lateral pterygoid plate is to
   A. retrude (retract) the mandible
   B. elevate the soft palate
   C. protrude (protract) the mandible
   D. tense the soft palate
   E. elevate the mandible

5. After entering the submandibular triangle, the lingual artery passes immediately deep to which of the following muscles?
   A. genioglossus
   B. anterior belly of the digastric
   C. mylohyoid
   D. hyoglossus
   E. styloglossus

6. A tumor infiltrating the foramen ovale might result in all of the following deficiencies **EXCEPT**
   A. paralysis of the tensor tympani muscle
   B. sensory loss to the skin of the lower lip
   C. anesthesia involving the temporomandibular joint
   D. motor loss to the stylohyoid muscle
   E. sensory loss to the lower premolars

7. Following a tonsillectomy, a patient noted loss of general sensation and taste from the posterior one-third of the tongue. It could be assumed that the injured nerve was a branch of the
   A. glossopharyngeal nerve
   B. facial nerve
   C. lingual nerve
   D. vagus nerve
   E. hypoglossal nerve

8. Pulsations felt at the lower border of the mandible just anterior to the masseter muscle are in the
   A. superficial temporal artery
   B. lingual artery
   C. maxillary artery
   D. transverse facial artery
   E. facial artery

9. The structure that lies parallel and immediately deep to the carotid sheath in the neck is the
   A. superior ramus of the ansa cervicalis
   B. trachea
   C. sympathetic trunk
   D. internal jugular vein
   E. vagus nerve

10. A severe blow to the side of the head could fracture which one of the following bones in the roof of the orbit?
    A. palatine
    B. maxilla
    C. frontal
    D. zygomatic
    E. lacrimal

11. The largest structure on the medial wall of the tympanic cavity is the
    A. fenestra vestibuli
    B. facial canal
    C. umbo
    D. promontory
    E. fenestra cochlea

12. The artery that accompanies the inferior alveolar nerve is a branch of the
    A. superficial temporal artery
    B. maxillary artery
    C. posterior auricular artery
    D. facial artery
    E. lingual artery

**13.** Sympathetic preganglionic nerve fibers that are destined to supply the arteries of the head synapse in the
  A. ciliary ganglion
  B. superior cervical chain ganglion
  C. submandibular ganglion
  D. inferior cervical chain ganglion
  E. pterygopalatine ganglion

**14.** The muscle that rotates the muscular process of the arytenoid cartilage anteriorly, thus adducting the vocal folds, is the
  A. transverse arytenoid
  B. posterior cricoarytenoid
  C. lateral cricoarytenoid
  D. thyroarytenoid
  E. aryepiglottic

**15.** The medial wall of the pterygopalatine fossa is formed by which of the following bones?
  A. greater wing of sphenoid
  B. lateral pterygoid plate
  C. medial pterygoid plate
  D. maxilla
  E. palatine

**16.** A severe infection that obstructs the middle meatus would affect drainage from each of the following sinuses **EXCEPT** the
  A. maxillary sinus
  B. frontal sinus
  C. nasolacrimal duct
  D. anterior ethmoid air cells
  E. middle ethmoid air cells

**17.** The submandibular gland receives its primary blood supply from branches of which of the following arteries?
  A. facial
  B. lingual
  C. superior thyroid
  D. posterior auricular
  E. occipital

18. Damage to the posterior superior alveolar nerve would affect sensory innervation from the
    A. hard palate
    B. soft palate
    C. upper molars
    D. nasal mucosa
    E. mucosa of the floor of mouth

19. A complete anteroposterior cleft of the hard palate would involve the
    A. sphenoid and zygomatic bones
    B. maxillary and frontal bones
    C. ethmoid and frontal bones
    D. palatine and maxillary bones
    E. palatine and ethmoid bones

20. A lesion of the lingual nerve immediately after it receives the chorda tympani nerve could result in each of the following **EXCEPT**
    A. loss of sublingual gland secretion
    B. sensory loss from lower teeth
    C. loss of taste from anterior two-thirds of the tongue
    D. loss of submandibular gland secretion
    E. sensory loss from mucosa on floor of mouth

21. The osseous labyrinth of the internal ear consists of the
    A. vestibule
    B. sacculus
    C. semicircular ducts
    D. utriculus
    E. cochlear duct

22. The nerve to the mylohyoid muscle is correctly described by each of the following **EXCEPT** that
    A. it contains fibers of the mandibular nerve
    B. it forms the mylohyoid groove on the mandible
    C. it innervates the anterior belly of the digastric muscle
    D. it enters the mandibular foramen
    E. it courses, in part, with the submental artery

**23.** Each of the following correctly describes relationships of the anterior scalene muscle **EXCEPT** that the
  **A.** phrenic nerve descends on its anterior surface
  **B.** thyrocervical trunk is lateral to the muscle
  **C.** brachial plexus passes posteriorly
  **D.** subclavian artery passes posteriorly
  **E.** suprascapular artery passes anteriorly

**24.** Difficulty in retraction of the mandible would indicate damage to the
  **A.** lateral pterygoid muscle
  **B.** masseter muscle
  **C.** mylohyoid muscle
  **D.** medial pterygoid muscle
  **E.** posterior fibers of the temporalis muscle

**25.** A lesion that compresses the neural contents within the right jugular foramen might result in
  **A.** loss of pain from the anterior two-thirds of the tongue
  **B.** inability to protrude the tongue
  **C.** sensory loss from skin overlying the zygomatic bone
  **D.** inability to elevate the soft palate
  **E.** inability to turn the chin upward and to the left

**26.** A ligature occluding the external carotid artery just distal to the lingual artery would probably stop the flow of blood to each of the following **EXCEPT** the
  **A.** inferior alveolar artery
  **B.** superficial temporal artery
  **C.** infraorbital artery
  **D.** middle meningeal artery
  **E.** superior laryngeal artery

**27.** The palatine tonsil lies between which of the following pairs of muscles?
  **A.** palatoglossus and styloglossus
  **B.** superior pharyngeal constrictor and stylopharyngeus
  **C.** stylopharyngeus and styloglossus
  **D.** palatopharyngeus and palatoglossus
  **E.** palatoglossus and stylopharyngeus

**28.** A tonsillar abscess may extend posteriorly through the posterior pharyngeal wall into the
   **A.** pleural cavity
   **B.** anterior triangle of the neck
   **C.** suprasternal space
   **D.** pharyngeal tonsil
   **E.** retropharyngeal space

**29.** After exiting the stylomastoid foramen, the facial nerve is correctly described by each of the following **EXCEPT**
   **A.** it innervates the posterior belly of the digastric and stylohyoid muscles
   **B.** it courses superficial to the retromandibular vein
   **C.** it innervates the muscle that provides tone to the cheek
   **D.** it innervates the submandibular and sublingual glands
   **E.** it innervates the muscles that elevate the upper lip

**30.** Ligation of the subclavian artery would affect the blood supply to each of the following **EXCEPT** the
   **A.** first intercostal space
   **B.** floor of the mouth
   **C.** trapezius muscle
   **D.** dorsal muscles of the scapula
   **E.** thyroid gland

**31.** Each of the following nerves conveys either preganglionic or postganglionic fibers to the parotid gland **EXCEPT** the
   **A.** lesser petrosal
   **B.** nerve of the pterygoid canal
   **C.** glossopharyngeal
   **D.** tympanic
   **E.** auriculotemporal

**32.** The superficial (investing) layer of the cervical fascia encloses which one of the following muscles?
   **A.** anterior scalene
   **B.** middle scalene
   **C.** sternohyoid
   **D.** sternocleidomastoid
   **E.** levator scapulae

**33.** Cell bodies of parasympathetic preganglionic neurons to the glands of the hard palate are located in the
   **A.** pterygopalatine ganglion
   **B.** otic ganglion
   **C.** geniculate ganglion
   **D.** submandibular ganglion
   **E.** brain

**34.** If a patient presented with a permanently dilated pupil, which one of the following nerves could be assumed to be involved?
   **A.** optic
   **B.** sympathetic trunk
   **C.** ophthalmic
   **D.** oculomotor
   **E.** facial

**35.** The inferior root (ramus) of the ansa cervicalis contains nerve fibers derived from the
   **A.** first and second cervical spinal nerves
   **B.** second and third cervical spinal nerves
   **C.** third and fourth cervical spinal nerves
   **D.** first, second, and third cervical spinal nerves
   **E.** hypoglossal nerve

**36.** When a patient attempts protrusion of the tongue, the tongue deviates to the right. This would indicate damage to which of the following nerves?
   **A.** right glossopharyngeal
   **B.** left accessory
   **C.** right hypoglossal
   **D.** left hypoglossal
   **E.** right lingual

**37.** Each of the following is related to the walls of the laryngeal part of the pharynx **EXCEPT** the
   **A.** piriform recess
   **B.** cricoid cartilage
   **C.** inferior pharyngeal constrictor muscle
   **D.** arytenoid cartilage
   **E.** palatine tonsil

---

**DIRECTIONS (Questions 38–51):** Each group of questions below consists of five lettered headings followed by a list of numbered words or statements. For each numbered word or statement, select the **one** lettered heading that is most closely associated with it. Each lettered heading may be selected once, more than once, or not at all.

---

**Questions 38–42:** Nerve function.

- **A.** Nasopalatine nerve
- **B.** Chorda tympani nerve
- **C.** Greater petrosal nerve
- **D.** Lesser petrosal nerve
- **E.** Deep petrosal nerve

38. Conveys postganglionic neurons that course through the pterygoid canal and have their cell bodies located in the superior cervical ganglion

39. Conveys impulses for taste from the anterior two-thirds of the tongue

40. Supplies sensory fibers from the anterior one-third of the hard palate

41. Contains parasympathetic preganglionic neurons that synapse in the pterygopalatine ganglion

42. Contains parasympathetic preganglionic neurons that synapse in the submandibular ganglion

**Questions 43–47:** Structures that traverse the foramina of the skull.

- **A.** Foramen ovale
- **B.** Foramen rotundum
- **C.** Petrotympanic fissure
- **D.** Superior orbital fissure
- **E.** Internal acoustic meatus

43. Mandibular nerve

44. Facial nerve

**45.** Maxillary nerve

**46.** Chorda tympani

**47.** Ophthalmic nerve

**Questions 48–51:** Nerve function.

    **A.** Internal branch of the superior laryngeal nerve
    **B.** External branch of the superior laryngeal nerve
    **C.** Glossopharyngeal nerve
    **D.** Inferior laryngeal nerve
    **E.** Facial nerve

**48.** Supplies sensory fibers from the mucosa of the piriform recess

**49.** Innervates a muscle that elevates the pharynx

**50.** Innervates the cricothyroid muscle

**51.** Provides sensory fibers form the mucosa of the larynx inferior to the vocal folds

---

**DIRECTIONS Questions 52–60:** For each of the following figures there is a list of numbered statements that describe lettered structures on the figures. For each numbered statement, identify the lettered structure on the figure.

---

**Questions 52–56 (Figure 1):** Nerves of superficial face and neck.

**52.** Could be damaged following a fracture of the roof of the maxillary sinus

**53.** Fibers traverse the foramen ovale and mandibular foramen

**54.** Derives from the ventral rami of the second and third cervical spinal nerves

**55.** Supplies somatic sensation from the mucosa of the check

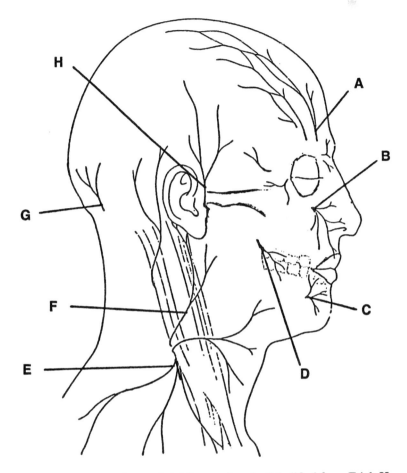

**Figure 1** Nerves of superficial face and neck. (Modified from Frick H, et al.: *Human Anatomy I.* Stuttgart: Georg Thieme Verlag, 1991).

**56.** Surrounds the middle meningeal artery in the infratemporal fossa and supplies sensory innervation from the temporomandibular joint

**Questions 57–60 (Figure 2):** Lateral view of neck.

**57.** Originates from the thyroid cartilage and is innervated by vagal fibers via the pharyngeal plexus

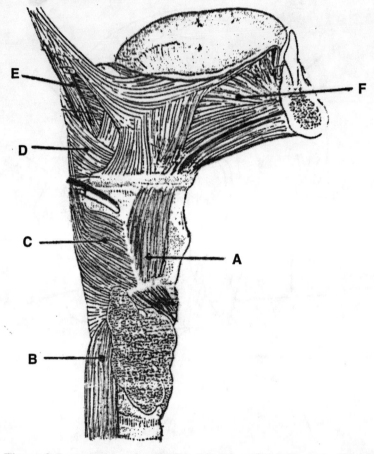

**Figure 2** Lateral view of neck. (Modified from Frick H, et al.: *Human Anatomy I. Stuttgart: Georg Thieme Verlag, 1991.*)

58. Is innervated by motor fibers from the cervical plexus

59. Forms the major muscular component of the tongue

60. Receives its primary motor innervation from the recurrent laryngeal nerve

# THE UPPER EXTREMITY

---

**DIRECTIONS Questions 61–88:** Each of the questions or incomplete statements below is followed by five suggested answers or completions. Select the **one** that is best in each case.

---

61. A penetrating knife wound to the posterior shoulder in the quadrangular space would damage the axillary nerve and the
    A. lateral thoracic artery
    B. anterior circumflex humeral artery
    C. subscapular artery
    D. superior thoracic artery
    E. posterior circumflex humeral artery

62. Following a hard blow to the anterior shoulder, a weakness of flexion of the arm at the shoulder joint would suggest damage to which of the following muscles?
    A. rhomboid major
    B. supraspinatus
    C. pectoralis minor
    D. biceps brachii
    E. teres major

63. The nerve most likely to be injured in fractures of the posterior humeral shaft is the
    A. median
    B. ulnar
    C. musculocutaneous
    D. radial
    E. axillary

64. An injury to the thoracodorsal nerve might affect which of the following movements?
    A. lateral rotation of the arm
    B. flexion of the arm
    C. rotation of the scapula
    D. elevation of the scapula
    E. extension of the arm

65. If the entire greater tubercle of the humerus was broken away as a result of an injury, which of the following movements of the humerus would be affected?
    A. flexion and abduction
    B. abduction and lateral rotation
    C. flexion and medial rotation
    D. extension and medial rotation
    E. flexion, abduction, and adduction

66. Each of the following muscles forms a boundary of the axilla EXCEPT the
    A. serratus anterior
    B. subscapularis
    C. pectoralis major
    D. supraspinatus
    E. pectoralis minor

67. Each of the following statements correctly describes the median nerve EXCEPT that it
    A. is derived from lateral and medial cords of the brachial plexus
    B. innervates muscles only in the forearm and hand
    C. is found deep to the axillary artery in the axilla
    D. travels within the neurovascular compartments of the arm
    E. crosses the brachial artery anteriorly at midarm level

68. When injecting an anesthesic agent into the subarachnoid space, which of the following is an important landmark for determining where to insert the needle through the skin of the back?
    A. iliac crest
    B. inferior angle of the scapula
    C. coccyx
    D. third sacral vertebra
    E. fourth lumbar vertebra

69. The superficial palmar arterial arch of the hand
    A. is located in the thenar compartment
    B. is distal to the deep palmar arterial arch

    **C.**  is deep to the tendons of the flexor digitorum profundus muscle

    **D.**  is formed primarily by the radial artery

    **E.**  courses with the deep branch of the ulnar nerve

**70.** Inability to flex the distal phalanx of the fourth and fifth digits of the hand would indicate damage to which of the following nerves?

    **A.**  radial

    **B.**  deep radial

    **C.**  median

    **D.**  anterior interosseous

    **E.**  ulnar

**71.** Lateral rotation of the humerus is a function of muscles innervated by which of the following nerves?

    **A.**  radial

    **B.**  suprascapular and axillary

    **C.**  axillary and dorsal scapular

    **D.**  accessory and thoracodorsal

    **E.**  thoracodorsal and dorsal scapular

**72.** The erector spinae muscle and other deep intrinsic muscles of the back are innervated by the

    **A.**  axillary nerve

    **B.**  dorsal rami of spinal nerves

    **C.**  accessory nerve

    **D.**  branches from the posterior cord of the brachial plexus

    **E.**  dorsal scapular nerve

**73.** An injury to the median nerve in the middle third of the arm would affect the

    **A.**  flexor carpi ulnaris muscle

    **B.**  adductor pollicis muscle

    **C.**  abductor digiti minimi muscle

    **D.**  abductor pollicis brevis muscle

    **E.**  extensor carpi radialis longus muscle

**74.** Damage to the anatomic snuffbox might be expected to injure the
   A. ulnar nerve
   B. median nerve
   C. ulnar artery
   D. radial artery
   E. capitate bone

**75.** If the brachial artery was ligated in the distal third of the arm, blood could still reach the forearm by means of each of the following arteries **EXCEPT** the
   A. ulnar
   B. superior ulnar collateral
   C. radial collateral
   D. middle collateral
   E. deep brachial

**76.** Each of these muscles would be paralyzed by a laceration of the origin of the deep branch of the ulnar nerve **EXCEPT** the
   A. abductor digiti minimi
   B. palmaris longus
   C. third and fourth lumbricals
   D. adductor pollicis
   E. dorsal interossei

**77.** A high-velocity bullet penetrates the posterior aspect of the shoulder and severely injures the origin of the posterior cord of the brachial plexus. Each of the following nerves might possibly be affected **EXCEPT** the
   A. upper subscapular
   B. axillary
   C. thoracodorsal
   D. radial
   E. medial pectoral

**78.** As a result of an injury to the ulnar nerve in the arm, all of the following changes in the hand will be noted **EXCEPT**
   A. a claw hand
   B. the thumb is strongly adducted
   C. loss of flexion of the distal interphalangeal joints of the fourth and fifth digits

    **D.** sensory loss on the little finger and one-half of the ring finger

    **E.** marked wasting in the hypothenar eminence

79. Sensory loss over the skin covering the dorsal surface of the thumb would indicate damage to the
    **A.** deep radial nerve
    **B.** superficial radial nerve
    **C.** anterior interosseous nerve
    **D.** median nerve
    **E.** ulnar nerve

80. Compression of the median nerve in the carpal tunnel deep to the flexor retinaculum could affect the functioning of each of the following muscles **EXCEPT** the
    **A.** second lumbrical
    **B.** opponens pollicis
    **C.** flexor pollicis brevis
    **D.** abductor pollicis brevis
    **E.** flexor carpi radialis

81. The dermatome on the medial aspect of the forearm and ulnar side of the hand is supplied by which spinal nerve?
    **A.** fifth cervical
    **B.** sixth cervical
    **C.** seventh cervical
    **D.** eighth cervical
    **E.** first thoracic

82. Damage to the median nerve in the arm would affect each of the following functions **EXCEPT**
    **A.** supination of the forearm
    **B.** pronation of the forearm
    **C.** flexion at the wrist
    **D.** abduction at the wrist
    **E.** flexion of the thumb

**83.** Inability to hold a piece of paper between the second and third digits would result from damage to the
   **A.** median nerve
   **B.** superficial radial nerve
   **C.** ulnar nerve
   **D.** anterior interosseous nerve
   **E.** radial nerve

**84.** Severe trauma directly to the central compartment of the palm could damage each of the following **EXCEPT** the
   **A.** lumbrical muscles
   **B.** tendons of the flexor digitorum profundus muscle
   **C.** radial artery
   **D.** ulnar bursa
   **E.** median nerve

**85.** The medial cord of the brachial plexus
   **A.** contains nerve fibers from spinal cord segments C-5, C-6, and C-7
   **B.** receives anterior division fibers from the posterior cord
   **C.** gives rise to the musculocutaneous nerve
   **D.** contains nerve fibers from spinal cord segments C-8 and T-1
   **E.** is posterior to the second part of the axillary artery

**86.** Concerning the distribution pattern of spinal nerves, each of the following is correct **EXCEPT** that
   **A.** only ventral rami form plexuses
   **B.** the spinal nerves exit the intervertebral foramen
   **C.** dorsal roots carry preganglionic sympathetic fibers
   **D.** dorsal and ventral rami carry motor and sensory fibers
   **E.** the dorsal rami supply the skin of the back and the deep, intrinsic muscles of the back

**87.** The cephalic vein is normally a tributary to the
   **A.** brachial vein
   **B.** axillary vein
   **C.** medial brachial vein

    **D.** subclavian vein
    **E.** lateral brachial vein

**88.** Pressure developing deep to the flexor retinaculum would affect each of the following **EXCEPT** the
    **A.** median nerve
    **B.** ulnar nerve
    **C.** tendons of the flexor digitorum superficialis muscle
    **D.** tendons of the flexor pollicis longus muscle
    **E.** tendons of the flexor digitorum profundus muscle

---

**DIRECTIONS (Questions 89–97):** Each group of questions below consists of lettered headings followed by a list of numbered words or statements. For each numbered word or statement, select the **one** lettered heading that is most closely associated with it. Each lettered heading may be selected once, more than once, or not at all.

---

**Questions 89–92:** Description of arteries.

    **A.** Radial artery
    **B.** Ulnar artery
    **C.** Brachial artery
    **D.** Deep brachial artery
    **E.** Superior ulnar collateral artery

**89.** Arises from brachial artery and accompanies the ulnar nerve in the arm

**90.** Gives origin to the common interosseous artery

**91.** Descends in the forearm deep to the flexor carpi ulnaris muscle

**92.** Gives lateral to the dorsal carpal arterial arch

**Questions 93–97:** Description of muscle innervation.

    **A.** Radial nerve
    **B.** Median nerve
    **C.** Ulnar nerve
    **D.** Musculocutaneous nerve
    **E.** Motor (recurrent) branch of median nerve

**93.** Flexor digitorum superficialis

**94.** Abductor pollicis brevis

**95.** Brachioradialis

**96.** Opponens pollicis

**97.** Triceps brachii

---

**DIRECTIONS (Questions 98–101):** In Figure 3, of the brachial plexus, identify the lettered parts described by the numbered statements below.

---

**98.** Damage to this nerve results in a winged scapula due to loss of function of the serratus anterior muscle

**99.** Innervates most of the anterior (preaxial) musculature of the forearm

**100.** Courses deep to the superior transverse scapular ligament

**101.** Damage to this nerve would result in wrist drop

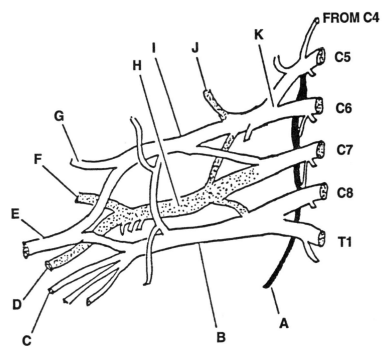

**Figure 3** Brachial plexus. (From Wilson JE. *Anatomy,* 9th ed. New York: Elsevier, 1991, p. 27.)

# THE LOWER EXTREMITY

**DIRECTIONS (Questions 102–137):** Each of the questions or incomplete statements below is followed by five answers or completions. Select the **one** that is best in each case.

102. Reduced blood supply to the lateral compartment of the leg results primarily from damage to the
   A. anterior tibial artery
   B. femoral artery
   C. lateral malleolar artery
   D. fibular artery
   E. peroneal artery

**103.** A patient enters the emergency room not being able to raise his foot. The nerve that is suspected to be damaged is the

    **A.** tibial

    **B.** common fibular

    **C.** obturator

    **D.** medial plantar

    **E.** lateral plantar

**104.** As the deep fibular nerve descends through the leg, it is joined by which one of the following arteries?

    **A.** popliteal

    **B.** sural

    **C.** posterior tibial

    **D.** middle genicular

    **E.** anterior tibial

**105.** The tibial collateral ligament (medial ligament of the knee) extends from the medial epicondyle of the femur to the

    **A.** lateral condyle of the tibia

    **B.** medial condyle of the tibia

    **C.** articular capsule

    **D.** neck of the fibula

    **E.** neck of the tibia

**106.** The powerful extension of the thigh required when one is standing from a sitting position is the function of the

    **A.** gluteus maximus muscle

    **B.** psoas major muscle

    **C.** iliacus muscle

    **D.** obturator externus muscle

    **E.** piriformis muscle

**107.** Loss of function of the muscles of the posterior compartment of the leg and the sole of the foot is associated with paralysis of the

    **A.** tibial nerve

    **B.** common fibular nerve

    **C.** superficial fibular nerve

    **D.** deep fibular nerve

    **E.** femoral nerve

**108.** The muscles of the posterior compartment of the thigh receive blood supply primarily by branches of the
   A. popliteal artery
   B. deep femoral artery
   C. superior gluteal artery
   D. inferior gluteal artery
   E. femoral artery

**109.** A significant weakness in adduction of the thigh would involve each of the following muscles **EXCEPT** the
   A. gluteus medius
   B. pectineus
   C. gracilis
   D. adductor magnus
   E. adducton brevis

**110.** All of the following statements describe the sartorius muscle **EXCEPT**
   A. it is innervated by the femoral nerve
   B. it arises from the anterior superior spine of the ilium
   C. it inserts on the lateral surface of the tibia
   D. it forms the lateral border of the femoral triangle
   E. its contraction produces flexion, abduction, and lateral rotation

**111.** Lateral rotation of the thigh involves each of the following muscles **EXCEPT** the
   A. gluteus maximus
   B. quadratus femoris
   C. gluteus minimus
   D. superior gemellus
   E. piriformis

**112.** Which of the following structures passes through the lesser sciatic foramen?
   A. piriformis muscle
   B. inferior gluteal nerve
   C. obturator internus muscle
   D. superior gluteal nerve
   E. sciatic nerve

113. Each of the following statements relating to the femoral sheath is true **EXCEPT** that
    A. it encloses the proximal portions of the femoral artery and vein
    B. it is formed by the tranversalis fascia
    C. the femoral nerve is lateral to the femoral sheath
    D. the inguinal ligament is anterior to the femoral sheath
    E. it is divided into three compartments with the femoral artery being located in the femoral canal

114. Coursing from the femoral triangle into the adductor canal of the thigh is the
    A. femoral artery
    B. femoral vein
    C. deep femoral artery
    D. saphenous nerve
    E. femoral nerve

115. The biceps femoris muscle has a dual innervation derived from which of the following pairs of nerves?
    A. femoral and obturator
    B. obturator and tibial
    C. tibial and common fibular
    D. femoral and common fibular
    E. tibial and femoral

116. A weakness in inversion of the foot would result from damage to which of the following muscles?
    A. flexor hallucis brevis
    B. flexor digitorum brevis
    C. tibialis anterior
    D. fibularis longus
    E. extensor digitorum brevis

117. Damage to the obturator nerve on the lateral wall of the pelvis would affect the function of each of the following muscles **EXCEPT** the
    A. sartorius
    B. gracilis
    C. adductor longus
    D. pectineus
    E. adductor magnus

**118.** Each of the following structures is located in the posterior compartment of the leg **EXCEPT** the
   **A.** posterior tibial artery
   **B.** soleus muscle
   **C.** flexor digitroum longus muscle
   **D.** tibial nerve
   **E.** medial plantar artery

**119.** Ligation of the posterior tibial artery at its origin would involve all of the following branches **EXCEPT** the
   **A.** dorsalis pedis artery
   **B.** lateral plantar artery
   **C.** plantar arterial arch
   **D.** fibular artery
   **E.** medial plantar artery

**120.** Which of the following muscles would lose innervation if the tibial nerve was sectioned at the level of the medial malleolus?
   **A.** tibialis posterior
   **B.** flexor digitorum longus
   **C.** plantaris
   **D.** flexor hallucis longus
   **E.** extensor hallucis longus

**121.** Cutaneous sensory loss as a result of damage to the tibial nerve in the popliteal fossa would be limited to the
   **A.** medial side of the leg
   **B.** dorsal surface of the foot
   **C.** anterior surface of the leg
   **D.** dorsum of the big toe only
   **E.** most of the heel and sole

**122.** The iliotibial tract receives tendinous reinforcement from the
   **A.** tensor fasciae latae muscle
   **B.** gluteal medius muscle
   **C.** inguinal ligament
   **D.** sacrotuberous ligament
   **E.** gluteus minimus muscle

**123.** The inferior gluteal nerve is a postaxial branch of the sacral plexus with the fibers from
    **A.** L-3, L-4, and L-5
    **B.** L-4, L-5, and S-1
    **C.** L-5, S-1, and S-2
    **D.** S-1, S-2, and S-3
    **E.** S-2, S-3, and S-4

**124.** The superior boundary (base) of the femoral triangle is formed by the
    **A.** sartorius muscle
    **B.** adductor longus muscle
    **C.** inguinal ligament
    **D.** pubic tubercle
    **E.** pectincus muscle

**125.** The superficial muscles of the posterior compartment of the leg insert on which of the following bones?
    **A.** talus
    **B.** navicular
    **C.** calcaneus
    **D.** tibia
    **E.** fibula

**126.** The lateral intermuscular septum of the thigh separates which of the following muscles?
    **A.** adductor longus and gracilis
    **B.** semitendinosus and gracilis
    **C.** psoas major and pectineus
    **D.** vastus lateralis and biceps femoris
    **E.** vastus lateralis and semitendinosus

**127.** A crushing blow that damages the anterior inferior iliac spine would damage the origin of the
    **A.** biceps femoris muscle
    **B.** pectineus muscle
    **C.** rectus femoris muscle
    **D.** tensor fasciae latae muscle
    **E.** psoas major muscle

**128.** Damage to the medial plantar nerve would affect each of the following muscles **EXCEPT** the
  **A.** quadratus plantae
  **B.** abductor hallucis
  **C.** flexor digitorum brevis
  **D.** flexor hallucis brevis
  **E.** first lumbrical

**129.** The roof of the adductor canal is formed by the
  **A.** rectus femoris muscle
  **B.** adductor longus muscle
  **C.** vastus medialis muscle
  **D.** sortorius muscle
  **E.** fascia lata

**130.** The femoral vessels enter the popliteal fossa through a hiatus in which one of the following muscles?
  **A.** adductor longus
  **B.** gracilis
  **C.** adductor magnus
  **D.** vastus medialis
  **E.** rectus femoris

**131.** The plantar arterial arch is formed by the lateral plantar artery and the
  **A.** medial plantar artery
  **B.** anterior tibial artery
  **C.** posterior tibial artery
  **D.** deep plantar artery
  **E.** fibular artery

**132.** The primary weight support function at the ankle joint is provided by which of the following bones?
  **A.** fibula and talus
  **B.** fibula and tibia
  **C.** tibia and calcaneus
  **D.** calcaneus and navicular
  **E.** tibia and talus

**133.** Loss of extension of the knee would result from damage to the
   **A.** femoral nerve
   **B.** tibial nerve
   **C.** tibial and common fibular nerves
   **D.** obturator and femoral nerves
   **E.** obturator nerve

**134.** Each of the following is correct concerning the femoral nerve **EXCEPT** that it
   **A.** enters the thigh lateral to the femoral sheath
   **B.** supplies motor nerves to most of the muscles of the anterior compartment of the thigh
   **C.** lies medial to the femoral artery in the femoral triangle
   **D.** has no motor branches below the knee
   **E.** supplies cutaneous branches to the medial surface of the leg

**135.** The superior lateral border of the popliteal fossa is formed by the
   **A.** semitendinosus and semimembranosus muscles
   **B.** biceps femoris muscle
   **C.** adductor longus muscle
   **D.** adductor magnus muscle
   **E.** gastrocnemius muscle

**136.** This nerve supplies the following muscles: adductor hallucis, abductor hallucis, abductor digiti minimi, flexor digiti minimi brevis, and the lateral three lumbricals
   **A.** anterior tibial nerve
   **B.** deep fibular nerve
   **C.** sural nerve
   **D.** medial plantar nerve
   **E.** lateral plantar nerve

**137.** Muscles that flex the leg include each of the following **EXCEPT** the
   **A.** biceps femoris
   **B.** rectus femoris
   **C.** semimembranosus
   **D.** gracilis
   **E.** semitendinosus

DIRECTIONS (Questions 138–140): The group of questions below consists of five lettered headings followed by a list of numbered words or statements. For each numbered word or statement, select the **one** lettered heading that is most closely associated with it. Each lettered heading may be selected once, more than once, or not at all.

    **A.** Iliopsoas muscle
    **B.** Gluteus minimus muscle
    **C.** Quadratus femoris muscle
    **D.** Gluteus maximus muscle
    **E.** Adductor magnus muscle

**138.** Originates from the ischial tuberosity and is a strong lateral rotator of the thigh

**139.** Functions as a strong flexor of the thigh

**140.** Functions as a medial rotator of the thigh and is an important muscle in locking the hip joint during walking

# THE THORAX

DIRECTIONS (Questions 141–168): Each of the questions or incomplete statements below is followed by five suggested answers or completions. Select the **one** that is best in each case.

**141.** The lateral boundary of the superior mediastinum is the
    **A.** lateral border of the sternum
    **B.** T-1 to T-4 vertebrae
    **C.** roots of the lungs
    **D.** sternal angle
    **E.** mediastinal pleura

**142.** Trauma to the sternocostal surface of the heart would most likely damage the
   **A.** right atrium
   **B.** right ventricle
   **C.** left ventricle
   **D.** right auricle
   **E.** left atrium

**143.** When removing the right lung, the surgeon has to be careful to protect which of the following structures passing posterior to the root of the lung?
   **A.** hemiazygos vein
   **B.** right vagus nerve
   **C.** right phrenic nerve
   **D.** thoracic aorta
   **E.** right recurrent laryngeal nerve

**144.** The coronary sinus receives each of the following vessels **EXCEPT** the
   **A.** great cardiac vein
   **B.** middle cardiac vein
   **C.** anterior cardiac vein
   **D.** small cardiac vein
   **E.** posterior vein of the left ventricle

**145.** A tumor involving the fifth to twelfth thoracic vertebrae could affect each of the following structures in the posterior mediastinum **EXCEPT** the
   **A.** thoracic duct
   **B.** phrenic nerve
   **C.** azygos vein
   **D.** descending aorta
   **E.** esophagus

**146.** The brachiocephalic veins usually receive venous blood directly from each of the following **EXCEPT** the
   **A.** subclavian vein
   **B.** internal jugular vein

**C.** external jugular vein
**D.** inferior thyroid vein
**E.** internal thoracic vein

**147.** Each of the following is related to the lumen of the right ventricle **EXCEPT** the
    **A.** interventricular septum
    **B.** trabeculae carneae
    **C.** bicuspid valve
    **D.** anterior papillary muscle
    **E.** septomarginal band

**148.** The greater splanchnic nerve contains nerve fibers derived from each of the following spinal nerves **EXCEPT**
    **A.** T-5
    **B.** T-12
    **C.** T-9
    **D.** T-7
    **E.** T-8

**149.** The left coronary artery bifurcates into the circumflex branch and the
    **A.** left marginal branch
    **B.** left ventricular branch
    **C.** anterior interventricular branch
    **D.** right marginal branch
    **E.** posterior interventricular branch

**150.** A patient undergoing a heart attack usually experiences excruciating pain running down the left upper extremity. This referred pain is relayed by the
    **A.** left recurrent laryngeal nerve
    **B.** left vagus nerve
    **C.** left phrenic nerve
    **D.** left intercostobrachial nerve
    **E.** left musculocutaneous nerve

**151.** Dissection in the coronary sulcus (atrioventricular groove) of the heart would demonstrate each of the following **EXCEPT** the
  A. right coronary artery
  B. circumflex branch of the left coronary artery
  C. great cardiac vein
  D. middle cardiac vein
  E. coronary sinus

**152.** The structure immediately deep to the sternun in the superior mediastinum is the
  A. aortic arch
  B. left brachiocephalic vein
  C. left common carotid artery
  D. right common carotid artery
  E. phrenic nerve

**153.** Each of the following arteries is a branch of the descending thoracic aorta **EXCEPT** the
  A. posterior intercostal
  B. esophageal
  C. bronchial
  D. left subclavian
  E. superior phrenic

**154.** Nerve fibers in the greater, lesser, and least splanchnic nerves are
  A. preganglionic sympathetic fibers
  B. postganglionic sympathetic fibers
  C. a mixture of pre- and postganglionic parasympathetic fibers
  D. preganglionic parasympathetic fibers
  E. postganglionic parasympathetic fibers

**155.** The spinal nerves of the thoracic and upper lumbar regions are unique in that they possess
  A. dorsal primary rami
  B. white rami communicantes
  C. gray rami communicantes
  D. dorsal roots of spinal nerves
  E. dorsal root ganglia

**156.** Within the superior mediastinum, the anterior surface of the esophagus is in a contact with the
   A. anterior longitudinal ligament of the vertebral column
   B. thoracic duct
   C. trachea
   D. thymus
   E. arch of the aorta

**157.** The thoracic duct is correctly described by each of the following **EXCEPT**
   A. it is the largest lymphatic channel in the body
   B. it arises in a dilatation known as the cisterna chyli within the abdomen
   C. it returns to the bloodstream lymph from all of the body below the diaphragm and from the left half of the body above the diaphragm
   D. it courses through the posterior mediastinum between the aorta and the azygos vein
   E. it diverges in the superior mediastinum to the right side of the esophagus toward the right superior aperture of the neck

**158.** On the diaphragmatic surface of the heart, the posterior interventricular sulcus separates which of the following chambers?
   A. right ventricle-right atrium
   B. left venticle-left atrium
   C. left atrium-right atrium
   D. left ventricle-right ventricle
   E. left venticle-right atrium

**159.** Parts of the parietal pleura are described by each of the following terms **EXCEPT**
   A. diaphagmatic
   B. cervical
   C. costal
   D. mediastinal
   E. basal

**160.** A myocardial infarct that damages the heart muscle in the anterior two-thirds of the interventricular septum would result primarily from occlusion of the
A. posterior interventricular artery
B. marginal branch of the right coronary artery
C. marginal branch of the left coronary artery
D. anterior interventricular artery
E. circumflex branch of the left coronary artery

**161.** Which one of the following structures in the posterior mediastinum is found immediately posterior to the left atrium and pericardium?
A. esophagus
B. vagus nerves
C. azygos vein
D. thoracic duct
E. right pulmonary artery

**162.** Each of the following statements correctly describes the costodiaphragmatic recess **EXCEPT**
A. it is an inferior extension of the pleural cavity
B. it represents an area where the costal and diaphragmatic layers of parietal pleura can come into apposition with each other
C. it is a subcompartment of the thoracic cavity
D. in quiet respiration, it is usually found deep to the eighth and ninth intercostal spaces in the midaxillary line
E. it contains a thin film of serous fluid

**163.** The most superior structure at the root of the left lung is the
A. pulmonary artery
B. superior pulmonary vein
C. primary bronchus
D. inferior pulmonary vein
E. azygos vein

**164.** The horizontal fissure of the right lung separates the
A. superior and middle lobes
B. superior and inferior lobes
C. inferior and middle lobes

**D.** superior lobe from the cardiac notch
**E.** superior lobe and lingula

165. Each of the following is found at the horizontal plane of the sternal angle **EXCEPT** the
   **A.** superior termination of the fibrous pericardium
   **B.** intervertebral disk between the fourth and fifth thoracic vertebrae
   **C.** beginning and termination of the aortic arch
   **D.** bifurcation of the trachea
   **E.** bifurcation of the brachiocephalic artery into the right subclavian and right common carotid arteries

166. The part of the rib that articulates with the transverse process of the vertebra is the
   **A.** superior articular facet
   **B.** inferior articular facet
   **C.** tubercle articular facet
   **D.** angle
   **E.** neck

167. The superior vena cava could be damaged by a stab wound deep to the
   **A.** right first costal cartilage
   **B.** right fourth costal cartilage
   **C.** right sternoclavicular joint
   **D.** left second costal cartilage
   **E.** left sternoclavicular joint

168. A stab wound through the thoracic wall deep to the fourth intercostal space on the right side of the sternum would first puncture the
   **A.** superior vena cava
   **B.** right brachiocephalic vein
   **C.** left brachiocephalic vein
   **D.** brachiocephalic trunk
   **E.** right atrium

**DIRECTIONS (Questions 169–185):** Each group of questions below consists of five lettered headings or an illustration with lettered structures, followed by a list of numbered words or statements. For each numbered word or statement, select the **one** lettered heading or structure that is most closely associated with it. Each lettered heading or structure may be selected once, more than once, or not at all.

A. Great cardiac vein
B. Right coronary artery
C. Small cardiac vein
D. Middle cardiac vein
E. Coronary sinus

**169.** Begins at the apex of the heart, ascends in the anterior interventricular sulcus, and terminates in the coronary sinus

**170.** Lies in the coronary sulcus and terminates in the right atrium

**171.** Accompanies the posterior interventricular artery and empties into the coronary sinus

**172.** Begins along the inferior margin of the heart, accompanies the right coronary artery, and empties into the coronary sinus

**Questions 173–177:** Identify the lettered structures shown in Figure 4.

**173.** Ascending aorta

**174.** Left ventricle

**175.** Apex of heart

**176.** Border of diaphragm

**177.** Right border of heart

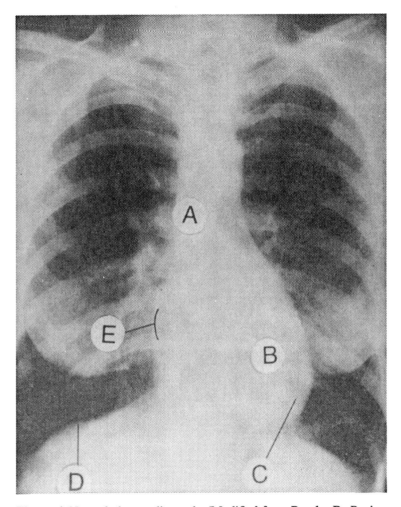

**Figure 4** Normal chest radiograph. (Modified from Pansky B: *Review of Gross Anatomy,* 5th ed. New York: McGraw-Hill, Inc, 1984.)

**Questions 178–185:** Identify the lettered structures shown in Figure 5.

**178.** Posterior interventricular artery

**179.** Right coronary artery

**180.** Circumflex artery

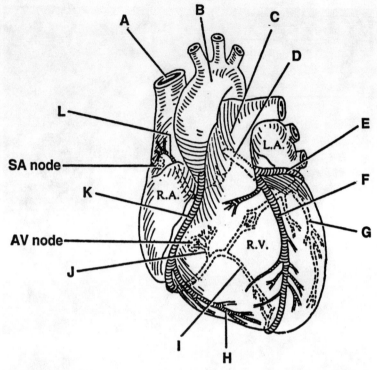

**Figure 5** Anterior view of heart. (Modified from Pansky B: *Review of Gross Anatomy,* 5th ed. New York: McGraw-Hill, Inc, 1984.)

**181.** Superior vena cava

**182.** Anterior interventricular artery

**183.** Pulmonary trunk

**184.** Aortic arch

**185.** Sinuatrial nodal artery

# THE ABDOMEN, PERINEUM, AND PELVIS

**DIRECTIONS (Questions 186–211):** Each of the questions or incomplete statements below is followed by five suggested answers or completions. Select the **one** that is best in each case.

**186.** The external abdominal oblique muscle and its fascia contribute to each of the following **EXCEPT** the
   A. lacunar ligament
   B. external spermatic fascia
   C. inguinal ligament
   D. anterior sheath of the rectus abdominis muscle
   E. falx inguinalis

**187.** A loss of bladder function would involve damage to parasympathetic preganglionic nerve fibers that have their cell bodies in the
   A. brain
   B. lateral horn of all thoracic spinal cord levels
   C. sacral spinal cord segments 2, 3, and 4
   D. lateral horn of the spinal cord at the upper lumbar levels
   E. lateral horn of all thoracic and upper three lumbar spinal cord levels

**188.** If the inferior mesenteric vein was ligated (tied off), blood from the sigmoid colon could still reach the liver because of anastomoses between the
   A. splenic and inferior mesenteric veins
   B. left colic and middle colic veins
   C. right colic and middle colic veins
   D. ileocolic and right colic veins
   E. left gastroepiploic and splenic veins

**189.** From which of the following sites is primary cancer most likely to metastasize to the lung by venous spread?
   A. ileum
   B. appendix
   C. kidney
   D. transverse colon
   E. sigmoid colon

**190.** During laparoscopic repair of an inguinal hernia, the following structure is used to establish the lateral boundary of the inguinal triangle
   A. inguinal ligament
   B. rectus abdominis muscle
   C. ischiopubic rami
   D. urogenital diaphragm
   E. inferior epigastric artery

**191.** Interruption of blood flow in the internal iliac artery would affect blood flow to each of the following **EXCEPT** the
   A. medial thigh muscles
   B. ductus deferens
   C. lower abdominal wall and rectus abdominis muscle
   D. urinary bladder
   E. rectum

**192.** An occlusion of the superior mesenteric artery would result in necrosis of each of the following **EXCEPT** the
   A. ascending colon
   B. rectum
   C. ileum
   D. cecum
   E. transverse colon

**193.** The posterior boundary of the epiploic foramen is formed by the
   A. duodenum
   B. lesser omentum
   C. stomach
   D. inferior vena cava
   E. transverse colon

**194.** The esophageal hiatus of the diaphragm transmits the esophagus and the
   A. superior phrenic artery
   B. thoracic duct
   C. vagal nerve trunks
   D. greater splanchnic nerve
   E. lesser splanchnic nerve

**195.** The hepatic portal vein is correctly described by each of the following **EXCEPT**
   A. it drains most of the venous blood from the gastrointestinal tract
   B. it forms by the confluence of the superior mesenteric and splenic veins
   C. it is located in the hepatoduodenal ligament
   D. it forms posterior to the head of the pancreas
   E. it forms the anterior border of the epiploic foramen

**196.** Cancer from the testis would most likely first metastasize to the
   A. lumbar nodes
   B. superficial inguinal nodes
   C. deep inguinal nodes
   D. internal iliac nodes
   E. external iliac nodes

**197.** The internal spermatic fascia is derived from the
   A. external abdominal oblique aponeurosis
   B. internal abdominal oblique aponeurosis
   C. transversus abdominis aponeurosis
   D. transversalis fascia
   E. peritoneum

**198.** Each of the following characterizes the levator ani muscle **EXCEPT**
   A. it forms the principal part of the pelvic diaphragm
   B. it provides an important support for pelvic viscera
   C. it arises from the inner surface of the superior ramus of the pubis
   D. it separates the floor of the pelvis from the ischioanal fossa
   E. it separates the superficial and deep inguinal spaces

**199.** Which one of the following arteries contributes to the blood supply of the pancreas?
   A. left gastroepiploic
   B. inferior mesenteric
   C. proper hepatic
   D. splenic
   E. left colic

**200.** Surgical damage to which one of the following arteries would affect blood supply to the suprarenal gland?
- **A.** renal
- **B.** gonadal
- **C.** superior mesenteric
- **D.** inferior mesenteric
- **E.** superior phrenic

**201.** The deep perineal space in the male contains each of the following **EXCEPT** the
- **A.** membranous urethra
- **B.** prostate gland
- **C.** bulbourethral glands
- **D.** deep transverse perineus muscle
- **E.** sphincter urethrae muscle

**202.** Each of the following characterizes the pudendal canal **EXCEPT**
- **A.** it is formed by a split in the obturator internus fascia
- **B.** it is located on the lateral wall of the ischioanal fossa
- **C.** it transmits the pudendal nerve
- **D.** it transmits the internal pudendal artery and vein
- **E.** it transmits lymphatics from the upper third of the rectum

**203.** The perineum receives its primary motor supply from which of the following nerves?
- **A.** pudendal
- **B.** inferior gluteal
- **C.** superior gluteal
- **D.** posterior femoral cutaneous
- **E.** ilioinguinal

**204.** Surgically, it is important to locate which one of the following structures located immediately posterior to the second part of the duodenum?
- **A.** transverse colon
- **B.** left lobe of the liver
- **C.** hilum of the right kidney
- **D.** superior mesenteric artery
- **E.** gallbladder

**205.** Postganglionic fibers from the celiac plexus and ganglia distribute with the
  A. middle colic artery
  B. left colic artery
  C. inferior pancreaticoduodenal artery
  D. left gastric artery
  E. right colic artery

**206.** Part of the anterior wall of the omental bursa is formed by the
  A. pancreas
  B. lesser omentum
  C. lienorenal ligament
  D. mesentery
  E. coronary ligament

**207.** All of the following statements correctly describe the deep inguinal ring **EXCEPT**
  A. it is a diverticulum of the transversalis fascia
  B. it is immediately lateral to the inferior epigastric artery
  C. it is the site of direct inguinal hernias
  D. it transmits the round ligament of the uterus
  E. it is reinforced anteriorly by fibers of the external abdominal oblique and internal abdominal oblique muscles

**208.** Pelvic splanchnic nerves are
  A. parasympathetics from the second, third and fourth sacral spinal cord segments
  B. sympathetics derived from the second, third and fourth sacral nerves
  C. direct branches of the sacral sympathetic trunk
  D. postganglionic sympathetic fibers ascending to the abdomen and thorax
  E. direct branches from the lumbar plexus to pelvic viscera

**209.** All of the following statements concerning the uterus are correct **EXCEPT**
- **A.** the broad ligament reflects from the posterior surface of the uterus to the rectum to form the rectouterine pouch
- **B.** the normal position of the uterus is described as anteverted and anteflexed
- **C.** the broad ligament extends from the anterior surface of the uterus onto the bladder, forming the vesicouterine pouch
- **D.** the round ligament connects the uterus to the ovary
- **E.** the uterine tubes enter the uterus in the superior border of the broad ligament

**210.** The crura of the clitoris or penis are attached to the
- **A.** transverse perineal ligament
- **B.** pubic symphysis
- **C.** ischial spines
- **D.** ischiopubic rami
- **E.** ischial tuberosities

**211.** The vagus nerve provides parasympathetic innervation to the gut as far as the
- **A.** duodenojejunal flexure
- **B.** ileocecal junction
- **C.** right colic flexure
- **D.** left colic flexure
- **E.** upper third of the rectum

**Questions 212–217:** Identify the lettered arteries of the stomach shown in Figure 6.

**212.** Courses along the superior border of the pancreas posterior to the body of the stomach

**213.** Branches from the abdominal aorta at the level of the first lumbar vertebra

**214.** Courses in the hepatoduodenal ligament to supply the liver

**215.** Courses in the gastrocolic ligament to supply the stomach and greater omentum

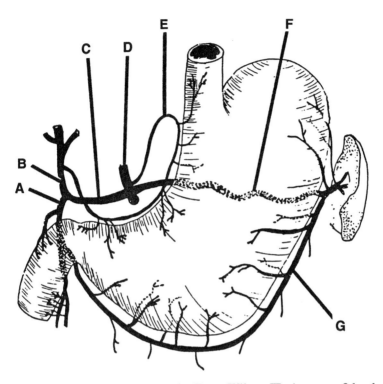

**Figure 6** Arteries of the stomach. (From Wilson JE. *Anatomy,* 9th ed. New York: Elsevier, 1991, p. 57.)

**216.** Courses in the lesser omentum and supplies the esophagus and stomach

**217.** Branches into the gastroduodenal and proper hepatic arteries

---

**DIRECTIONS (Questions 218–282):** Each of the case studies below is followed by numbered questions or incomplete statements. Select the **one** best lettered answer for each numbered question.

---

## Case Study I:

Upon admission to the hospital, a 40-year-old man was found to be acutely ill, with an elevated temperature, chills, vomiting, and intermittent delirium. He complained of headache, especially on the right side, and pain in the right eye. Approximately 2 weeks earlier, he had cut his upper lip while shaving, and a boil developed at the site.

Examination showed rigid neck muscles and marked swelling on the entire right side of the face. The upper lip was painful, extremely swollen, red, and oozing pus from several points. The right eyelid was swollen and there was right exophthalmos. The fundus of the right eye showed papilloedema and dilated retinal veins. No voluntary ocular muscles were functional in the right eye. Blood cultures were positive for *Staphylococcus aureus*. Leukocytosis indicated acute infection.

218. The most likely diagnosis is
    A. left transverse sinus thrombosis
    B. right cavernous sinus thrombosis
    C. superior sagittal sinus thrombosis
    D. hypophyseal tumor
    E. right transverse sinus thrombosis

219. Each of the following is true about the cavernous sinus **EXCEPT**
    A. it is drained by the superior and inferior petrosal sinuses
    B. the internal carotid artery lies in its lumen
    C. the superior ophthalmic vein is one of its principal tributaries
    D. the abducens nerve lies in its lateral wall
    E. it is located between the periosteal and meningeal dura mater

220. Each of the following provides venous drainage to the cavernous sinus **EXCEPT** the
    A. angular vein
    B. pterygoid plexus of veins
    C. straight sinus
    D. superior and inferior ophthalmic veins
    E. cerebral veins

221. The most vulnerable structure and often the first to be involved in cavernous sinus thrombosis is the
    A. oculomotor nerve
    B. abducens nerve
    C. ophthalmic division of the trigeminal nerve
    D. trochlear nerve
    E. maxillary division of the trigeminal nerve

**222.** Each of the following is enclosed in the tentorium cerebelli **EXCEPT** the
   A. straight sinus
   B. right transverse sinus
   C. superior petrosal sinus
   D. inferior petrosal sinus
   E. left transverse sinus

**223.** There was an inability to abduct the right eye and then look superiorly. This was due to damage to which of the following nerves?
   A. facial
   B. abducens
   C. oculomotor
   D. trochlear
   E. frontal

## Case Study II:

A 59-year-old man went to see his physician because of a swollen lower lip and a sore at the corner of the mouth. The medical history revealed that the lesion had been there for 6 years. Although it occasionally healed, it would sometimes break open and bleed.

   The physical examination showed an indurated, ulcerated area on the left lower lip at the angle of the mouth. Enlarged lymph nodes were palpable in the left carotid and submandibular triangles. A diagnosis of cancer of the lip with metastasis to the deep cervical nodes was confirmed by biopsy. Excision of the lip tumor was followed by a radical neck dissection.

**224.** Parts or all of the following can be sacrificed in a radical neck dissection **EXCEPT** the
   A. ansa cervicalis
   B. accessory nerve
   C. phrenic nerve
   D. submandibular gland
   E. internal jugular vein

**225.** Lymphatic flow from the corners of the lower lip usually drains first to the
    **A.** external jugular nodes
    **B.** submental nodes
    **C.** jugulo-omohyoid nodes
    **D.** parotid nodes
    **E.** submandibular nodes

**226.** Each of the following is closely related to the carotid sheath **EXCEPT** the
    **A.** vagus nerve
    **B.** internal carotid artery
    **C.** ansa cervicalis
    **D.** external carotid artery
    **E.** internal jugular vein

**227.** The structure that is located deep to the hyoglossus muscle in the submandibular triangle is the
    **A.** hypoglossal nerve
    **B.** lingual artery
    **C.** submandibular duct
    **D.** submandibular ganglion
    **E.** lingual nerve

**228.** Each of the following is related to the cervical visceral compartment **EXCEPT** the
    **A.** prevertebral fascia
    **B.** buccopharyngeal fascia
    **C.** trachea, larynx, pharynx
    **D.** thyroid gland
    **E.** pretracheal fascia

## Case Study III:

A 50-year-old dock worker tripped over cables and sprawled forward with his head turned to the right. He fell heavily, striking the deck on his left side, separating the head and shoulder.

On examination, the left arm was seen to hang limply at the side with the forearm pronated so that the palm was facing backward in the "waiter's tip" position. Abduction and lateral rotation at the shoulder joint were impossible, as was flexion at the elbow. Supination was weak. There was sensory loss on the lateral side of the patient's arm and forearm.

229. The most likely diagnosis is
   A. carpal tunnel syndrome
   B. Erb-Duchenne paralysis
   C. Volkman's contracture
   D. Klumpke's paralysis
   E. Dupuytren's contracture

230. The most probable cause of the arm limpness in this case is damage to the
   A. middle trunk of the brachial plexus
   B. lower roots of the brachial plexus
   C. upper roots of the brachial plexus
   D. spinal cord
   E. medial cord of the brachial plexus

231. The loss of flexion of the elbow resulted from damage to the
   A. axillary nerve
   B. thoracodorsal nerve
   C. long thoracic nerve
   D. musculocutaneous nerve
   E. median nerve

232. Axons in the superior trunk of the brachial plexus derive from which spinal cord levels?
   A. C-4, C-5, C-6
   B. C-5, C-6
   C. C-7, C-8
   D. C-8, T-1
   E. C-7, C-8, T-1

233. Axons in the musculocutaneous nerve derive from spinal cord levels
   A. C-5, C-6, C-7
   B. C-8, T-1
   C. C-4, C-5
   D. C-5, C-6
   E. C-7, C-8

**234.** This muscle is a powerful supinator and flexor at the elbow
   A. biceps brachii
   B. coracobrachialis
   C. brachialis
   D. anconeus
   E. triceps

**235.** Strong abductors at the shoulder joint are the
   A. teres major and infraspinatus muscles
   B. subscapularis and teres major muscles
   C. pectoralis major and bicep brachii muscles
   D. infraspinatus and teres minor muscles
   E. deltoid and supraspinatus muscles

**236.** These nerves derive from the posterior cord of the brachial plexus and innervate the most powerful medial rotator of the humerus
   A. upper and lower subscapular nerves
   B. suprascapular and dorsal scapular nerves
   C. thoracodorsal and long thoracic nerves
   D. medial and lateral pectoral nerves
   E. axillary and thoracodorsal nerves

**237.** The rotator (articular) cuff includes each of the following muscles **EXCEPT** the
   A. infraspinatus
   B. deltoid
   C. subscapularis
   D. teres minor
   E. supraspinatus

## Case Study IV:

A 35-year-old man presented to the emergency room complaining of severe pain and redness in his swollen left hand. He stated that he had cut his left index finger 2 weeks previously, with progressive pain since that time.

Examination revealed the cut on the dorsum of the proximal phalanx of his left index finger. The entire dorsum of the left hand was swollen. There was tenderness over the flexor surface of the left index finger. Lymph nodes in the left axilla were swollen and the patient's temperature was 101°F.

**238.** The most likely diagnosis is
- **A.** extensor expansion infection of the left index finger
- **B.** carpal tunnel syndrome and infection
- **C.** digital fibrous and synovial sheath infection of the left index finger
- **D.** infection in the ulnar bursa
- **E.** infection in the midpalmar space

**239.** The palm is not swollen but the dorsum is because the
- **A.** flexor tendons are on the dorsum of the hand
- **B.** extensor tendons have no synovial sheaths
- **C.** flexor tendons have no synovial sheaths
- **D.** the flexor retinaculum prevents swelling
- **E.** dense palmar aponeurosis prevents swelling in the palm

**240.** Infection of the flexor tendons and sheaths to the index finger would most likely spread first to the
- **A.** ulnar bursa
- **B.** thenar space
- **C.** anatomic snuffbox
- **D.** midpalmar space
- **E.** radial bursa

**241.** The radial bursa is occupied by the
- **A.** flexor digitorum profundus tendon
- **B.** adductor pollicis longus tendon
- **C.** lumbrical tendons
- **D.** flexor pollicis longus tendon
- **E.** flexor digitorum superficialis tendon

**242.** Each of the following groups of lymph nodes is directly involved in lymphatic drainage of the hand **EXCEPT** the
- **A.** mediastinal nodes
- **B.** cubital nodes
- **C.** pectoral nodes
- **D.** lateral axillary nodes
- **E.** central axillary nodes

## Case Study V:

A 26-year-old man lost control of his motorcycle on a gravel road. The cycle fell to the right, pinning the man's lower right limb between the bike and the road. There was severe pain and bleeding from the limb when the emergency medical team arrived.

Initial treatment and physical examination in the emergency room revealed a deep cut at the head of the fibula and a deep puncture wound in the midline of the calf of the leg. The neurologic examination indicated normal sensation from the dorsum of the foot except for loss of sensation from the skin between the first and second toes. There was significant loss of dorsiflexion at the ankle joint and loss of extension of the five toes. Plantar flexion, toe flexion, and eversion were normal. A normal pulse was felt on the dorsum of the foot, but was weak at the medial malleous.

243. The motor deficits observed during the neurologic examination would suggest damage to which of the following nerves?
    A. tibial
    B. common fibular
    C. deep fibular
    D. superficial fibular
    E. femoral

244. Each of the following muscles would be involved with either the loss of dorsiflexion or toe extension **EXCEPT** the
    A. fibularis longus
    B. extensor digitorum longus
    C. extensor hallucis longus
    D. tibialis anterior
    E. extensor hallucis brevis

245. The puncture wound on the middle of the posterior surface of the leg was the source of most of the bleeding. The primary source of the bleeding would most likely be the
    A. dorsalis pedis artery
    B. anterior tibial artery
    C. tibial artery
    D. femoral artery
    E. posterior tibial artery

**246.** The presence of sensation on the lateral side of the dorsum of the foot suggests that one of the following nerves was not damaged in the accident.

A. tibial
B. superficial fibular
C. deep fibular
D. lateral plantar
E. femoral

**247.** Which one of the following arteries was palpated to establish normal pulse distal to the extensor retinaculum on the dorsum of the foot?

A. posterior tibial
B. fibular
C. femoral
D. dorsalis pedis
E. medial plantar

## Case Study VI:

A 29-year-old man experienced extensive trauma to his left hip in a car accident. The initial examination indicated that there was significant general tissue damage to the nerves, vessels, and muscles surrounding the left hip joint and gluteal region. In addition, radiographs showed a fracture of the neck of the femur.

After 1 month of medical care and physical therapy, a neurologic examination showed that the left limb was externally (laterally) rotated and that there was difficulty in flexion at the knee joint, weakness in plantar flexion at the ankle joint, and general numbness on the posterior aspect of the calf of the leg. Radiographs concerned the physician because early signs of avascular necrosis of the femoral head were apparent.

**248.** The early stages of necrosis of the head of the femur observed after 1 month could result from damage to all of the following arteries supplying the head and neck of the femur **EXCEPT** the

A. medial circumflex femoral
B. lateral circumflex femoral
C. femoral
D. obturator
E. inferior gluteal

**249.** The loss of sensation on the posterior aspect of the calf of the leg resulted from compression of the
   A. tibial portion of the sciatic nerve
   B. obturator nerve
   C. femoral nerve
   D. posterior femoral cutaneous nerve
   E. saphenous nerve

**250.** Each of these muscles functions in internal (medial) rotation of the thigh at the hip joint **EXCEPT** the
   A. pectineus
   B. gracilis
   C. gluteus medius
   D. gluteus minimum
   E. sartorius

**251.** The externally (laterally) rotated thigh that was present 1 month after the accident would result from the loss of action of muscles that are innervated by which of the following pairs of nerves?
   A. common fibular and obturator
   B. superior gluteal and femoral
   C. femoral and tibial
   D. tibial and inferior gluteal
   E. obturator and superior gluteal

**252.** The significant reduction in knee flexion and plantar flexion at the ankle joint resulted from the loss of function of which of the following?
   A. superficial muscles of the calf and the hamstring muscles of the thigh
   B. anterior compartment muscles of the leg and quadriceps muscles of the thigh
   C. medial muscles of the thigh and deep muscles of the calf
   D. medial muscles of the thigh and quadriceps muscles of the thigh
   E. anterior compartment muscles of the leg and hamstring muscles of the thigh

## Case Study VII:

A 60-year-old man presented with symptoms of a constant, productive cough. Blood-tinged sputum had been noticed for several months. The patient complained of a heavy, uncomfortable feeling in the left chest, as well as shortness of breath. There had been significant weight loss, and recently the cough had begun keeping him awake at night.

The x-ray examination of the chest showed collapse of the left lower lobe. A bronchoscopic examination revealed a tumor in the left lower lobe bronchus. Biopsy confirmed it to be carcinoma. Biopsy of the deep cervical lymph nodes (supraclavicular lymph nodes) on both sides revealed that metastases had occurred bilaterally. A diagnosis of bronchogenic carcinoma was made. Involvement of the contralateral mediastinal nodes as well as the deep cervical nodes on both sides obviated surgery, and palliative treatment was begun. When the patient died after a few months, autopsy showed a cancerous tumor that had occluded the left lower lobe bronchus, penetrated the bronchus, and invaded the lung parenchyma. The remainder of the left lobe was collapsed and cancerous nodes were present in the hilus of both lungs and along the trachea. Metastases were present in the suprarenal glands and brain.

**253.** Enlarging, cancerous mediastinal lymph nodes could result in any of the following complications **EXCEPT**
   **A.** obstruction of the superior vena cava
   **B.** difficulty in swallowing (dysphagia)
   **C.** obstruction of the inferior vena cava
   **D.** hoarseness of the voice
   **E.** partial paralysis of the diaphragm

**254.** The metastasis of left lower lobe cancer differs from that in the right lobe in that the
   **A.** left superior broncomediastinal lymph nodes drain to those of the right side
   **B.** left inferior tracheobronchial lymph nodes drain to those of the right side
   **C.** right superior tracheobronchial lymph nodes commonly drain to those of the left side
   **D.** left posterior mediastinal lymph nodes drain bilaterally
   **E.** right inferior tracheobronchial nodes typically drain to those of the left side

**255.** The presence of cancer in which of the following lymph nodes verifies the diagnosis of metastatic carcinoma and precludes chest surgery?
A. bronchopulmonary nodes
B. pulmonary nodes
C. tracheobronchial nodes
D. paratracheal nodes
E. deep cervical (supraclavicular) nodes

**256.** During biopsy of the right cervical nodes, all of the following structures must be carefully avoided **EXCEPT** the
A. vagus nerve
B. phrenic nerve
C. thoracic duct
D. internal jugular vein
E. dome of the pleura (Sibson's fascia)

## Case Study VIII:

A 58-year-old man presented with a 2-year history of pain that would begin in the left shoulder and arm and then radiate to the sternum and mandible. The attacks of pain were increasing in frequency and were only relieved by rest.

The physical examination showed no involvement of the muscles, joints, or nerves in the involved areas. The heart was slightly enlarged on radiography. Based on the description of the pain and the age of the patient, a diagnosis of angina pectoris was made. Nitrites were given to dilate the coronary arteries and cardiac catheterization was proposed, with possible future coronary bypass surgery.

**257.** Pain afferents from the heart that were felt during the angina attacks synapse in the dorsal gray of spinal cord segments
A. T-1 to T4 or T5
B. T-8 to L-1
C. C-8 to T-3
D. T-1 to T-8
E. T-6 to T-8

**258.** Sensory cardiac nerves course in the
   A. dorsal roots of T-6 to T-8
   B. gray rami communicantes
   C. lower thoracic sympathetic chain ganglia
   D. ventral roots of T-6 to T-8
   E. white rami communicantes

**259.** The coronary arteries are constricted by
   A. postganglionic sympathetic nerves
   B. preganglionic and postganglionic fibers of the vagus nerve
   C. preganglionic and postganglionic sympathetic nerves
   D. preganglionic sympathetic nerves
   E. preganglionic fibers of the vagus and sympathetic nerves

**260.** The sinuatrial node is primarily innervated by the
   A. left vagus nerve
   B. right and left sympathetic preganglionic nerves
   C. left sympathetic postganglionic nerves
   D. right vagus nerve and right sympathetic nerves
   E. right and left vagus nerves

**261.** The cardiac catheterization revealed an area of occlusion of the circumflex branch of the left coronary artery. The damage to the heart would probably involve the
   A. left atrium and left ventricle
   B. right atrium and left ventricle
   C. left ventricle and interventricular septum
   D. apex of the heart
   E. right and left ventricles

# Case Study IX:

A 40-year-old male executive began to experience attacks of nausea and gnawing epigastric pain. When the stomach was empty, the pain worsened. Food intake and antacid gave some relief. On the day of his presentation, after a heavy lunch, the patient complained of excruciating pain in the abdomen and an ambulance was called.

Upon examination, the patient complained of agonizing epigastric pain. There was marked tenderness in the epigastrium. Temperature and blood pressure were normal. The past history and present events made a diagnosis of perforated ulcer (duodenal or gastric) likely and surgery was begun. When the abdomen was opened, fluid and particulate matter were found in the peritoneal cavity. Since there was no sign of an ulcer on the anterior wall of the stomach or duodenum, it was assumed that an ulcer on the posterior wall had perforated. When the omental bursa was opened, food particles and fluid were found. A perforated ulcer was found on the posterior wall of the body of the stomach. Laboratory examination revealed that it was not malignant, and the defect was closed.

262. Visceral pain from the stomach is transmitted through all of the following **EXCEPT** the
   A. white rami communicantes
   B. greater splanchnic nerves
   C. celiac ganglion
   D. spinal nerves
   E. least splanchnic nerve

263. Incision of which one of the following would not allow access to the omental bursa?
   A. transverse mesocolon
   B. hepatogastric ligament
   C. gastrolienal ligament
   D. falciform ligament
   E. hepatoduodenal ligament

264. Each of the following is related to the greater omentum **EXCEPT** the
   A. phrenicocolic ligament
   B. lienorenal ligament
   C. gastrocolic ligament
   D. gastrophrenic ligament
   E. gastrolienal ligament

265. Which one of these peritoneal ligaments is incorrectly matched with the blood vessel it contains?
   A. gastrocolic ligament-left gastroepiploic artery
   B. lesser omentum-right gastric artery
   C. gastrophrenic ligament-splenic artery
   D. transverse mesocolon-middle colic artery
   E. gastrolienal ligament-left gastroepiploic artery

**266.** The eroding ulcer on the posterior stomach wall is likely to first invade the

   **A.** pancreas
   **B.** liver
   **C.** duodenum
   **D.** transverse colon
   **E.** spleen

## Case Study X:

A 50-year-old, obese woman presented with severe pain in the right hypochondrium. She had had several such attacks, usually with nausea and vomiting. The attacks usually occurred after eating.

Examination showed rigidity and tenderness in the right hypochondriac region. Also on the right, there was pain around the side to the inferior angle of the scapula. The patient had an elevated white cell count and an elevated temperature. Multiple stones in the gallbladder and common bile duct were seen on the radiography. Surgery was scheduled.

**267.** Pain in the right hypochondrium that radiates to the scapular region suggests a diagnosis of

   **A.** appendicitis
   **B.** perforated ulcer
   **C.** kidney disease
   **D.** gallbladder disease
   **E.** pancreatitis

**268.** It would be difficult for a gallbladder infection to easily reach which one of the following viscera?

   **A.** liver
   **B.** third part of the duodenum
   **C.** cystic duct
   **D.** transverse colon
   **E.** first part of the duodenum

**269.** During removal of the gallbladder, which of the following arteries would need to be located in order to identify and ligate the cystic artery?
   **A.** right hepatic artery
   **B.** proper hepatic artery
   **C.** right gastric artery
   **D.** gastroduodenal artery
   **E.** left hepatic artery

**270.** Each one of the following correctly describes the common bile duct **EXCEPT**
   **A.** the posterior superior pancreaticoduodenal artery and vein spiral around the pancreatic portion of the duct
   **B.** it lies to the right of the proper hepatic artery in the right free margin of the hepatoduodenal ligament
   **C.** the common bile duct and pancreatic duct pass together through the wall of the second part of the duodenum
   **D.** descending posterior to the first part of the duodenum, it crosses the posterior surface of the head of the pancreas
   **E.** in the lesser omentum, it lies posterior to the portal vein

**271.** Which one of the following statements about the liver is false?
   **A.** the falciform ligament encloses the obliterated umbilical vein (ligamentum teres), which terminates in the left branch of the portal vein
   **B.** the coronary ligament reflects from the diaphragm as the right and left coronary and triangular ligaments
   **C.** the porta hepatis is the region of the entrance of the hepatic artery and hepatic vein and exit of the right and left hepatic bile ducts
   **D.** the fissure for the ligamentum venosum lodges the remains of the ductus venosus, which extends from the left branch of the portal vein to the left hepatic vein
   **E.** internal drainage of the intrahepatic ducts indicates that the right lobe includes the caudate lobe and the left lobe includes the quadrate lobe

## Case Study XI:

A 45-year-old man noticed a mass in his right inguinal region that had lasted for 3 or 4 months. Because of the development of pain and increased size of the lump over the previous 6 to 8 weeks, the patient made an appointment with his physician. During the examination, the physician determined that the mass was an inguinal hernia that had developed because of a weakened anterior abdominal wall resulting from years of manual factory labor. The hernia was corrected with surgery.

**272.** Which one of the following relationships would determine whether the hernia in the gut was an indirect inguinal hernia?
A. the hernia courses medial to the inferior epigastric artery
B. the hernia courses through the deep inguinal ring of the inguinal canal
C. the hernia passes through the inguinal (Hasselbach's) triangle
D. the hernia courses only through the superficial ring of the inguinal canal
E. the hernia courses through the posterior wall of the inguinal canal

**273.** Compression by the herniated gut of the nerve that lies on the external surface of the spermatic cord at the superficial inguinal ring would result in loss of
A. sensation from the dorsal surface of the penis
B. motor innervation to the rectus abdominis muscle at the level of the umbilicus
C. sensation from the anterior surface of the scrotum
D. motor function of the cremaster muscle
E. motor function to the bulbocavernosus muscle

**274.** The roof of the inguinal canal is formed by the internal abdominal oblique muscle and the
A. transversus abdominis muscle
B. transversalis fascia
C. external spermatic fascia
D. external abdominal oblique muscle
E. inguinal ligament

275. Which of the following structures would block herniation of a direct inguinal hernia through the medial aspect of the posterior wall of the inguinal canal?
    A. peritoneum
    B. inguinal ligament
    C. inferior epigastric artery
    D. lacunar ligament
    E. falx inguinalis

276. Visceral pain developing from the herniated gut would be conducted in nerve fibers contained in each of the following **EXCEPT** the
    A. pelvic splanchnic nerve
    B. greater splanchnic nerve
    C. lesser splanchnic nerve
    D. white rami communicantes
    E. thoracic spinal cord levels T-5 to T-12

## Case Study XII:

After noticing some abnormal vaginal bleeding that had occurred for several months and was not related to her normal menstrual cycle plus the recent development of pelvic pain over the previous few weeks, a 39-year-old woman visited her obstetrician and gynecologist. A cervical mass was suspected during the pelvic examination. A Pap smear was ordered and indicated abnormal cells. A biopsy confirmed a cervical malignancy. Computed tomography (CT) and magnetic resonance (MR) imaging indicated that the tumor had extended through the wall of the cervix. Surgery was scheduled immediately. Because positive cervical and uterine nodes were found during surgery, a radical hysterectomy and lymphadenectomy were performed.

277. Metastasis of cancer cells from the cervix would usually drain first into the
    A. superficial inguinal nodes
    B. deep inguinal nodes
    C. internal iliac nodes
    D. lumbar chain of nodes
    E. cisterna chyli

**278.** During the operation, the surgeon separates the two layers of the broad ligament to expose and ligate the uterine artery. Before ligating this artery, which one of the following structures located inferior to the uterine artery at the lateral side of the cervix has to be identified and protected?

    **A.** internal iliac artery
    **B.** pudendal nerve
    **C.** internal pudendal artery
    **D.** ureter
    **E.** coils of the ileum

**279.** Which one of the following structures is identified in the anterior layer of the broad ligament?

    **A.** round ligament
    **B.** ovarian ligament
    **C.** umbilical artery
    **D.** uterine tube
    **E.** tendinous arch of the levator ani muscle

**280.** Which one of the following pairs of structures must be protected while removing lymph nodes on the surface of the obturator internus muscle at the lateral pelvic wall?

    **A.** ureter and ovarian artery
    **B.** bladder and urethra
    **C.** obturator nerve and artery
    **D.** sciatic nerve and superior gluteal artery
    **E.** pudendal nerve and internal pudendal artery

**281.** As the surgeon identifies the ureter crossing the pelvic brim, it is clinically important to note that the ureter is immediately medial to and has to be separated from the

    **A.** aorta
    **B.** suspensory ligament of the ovary (infundibulopelvic ligament)
    **C.** ovary
    **D.** inferior vena cava
    **E.** uterine tube

**282.** If normal vascular anatomy is observed during surgery, the surgeon will attempt to preserve the first, large dorsal branch of the internal iliac (hypogastric) artery in order to maintain blood supply to which of the following muscles or muscle groups?
   **A.** adductor muscles of the thigh
   **B.** quadriceps femoris muscle of the thigh
   **C.** hamstring muscles of the thigh
   **D.** flexor muscles of the thigh
   **E.** gluteal muscles

# Gross Anatomy

## Answers and Comments

## THE HEAD AND NECK

**1. (E)**  The sphenoid bone contains the foramen rotundum, ovale, and spinosum. These foramina transmit the maxillary division of the 5th cranial nerve, the mandibular division of the 5th cranial nerve, and the middle meningeal artery, respectively. (**Ref. 2, p. 321**)

**2. (B)**  The four major groups of lymph nodes of the tongue (basal, marginal, central, and apical) drain directly or indirectly into the superior deep cervical lymph nodes situated along the course of the internal jugular vein. (**Ref. 2, p. 276**)

**3. (D)**  The middle meningeal artery passes through the foramen spinosum to enter the cranial cavity, where it becomes the principal artery of the dura mater. It is the largest branch of the first part of the maxillary artery. (**Ref. 2, p. 268**)

**4. (E)**  The medial pterygoid muscle has its origin mainly from the medial aspect of the lateral pterygoid plate. Its primary action is to elevate the mandible. It also assists in lateral movements of the mandible. (**Ref. 2, p. 260**)

**5. (D)** The lingual artery arises from the external carotid artery and, after a short course in the carotid triangle, disappears deep to the posterior border of the hyoglossus muscle. It supplies the tissue in the floor of the oral cavity. **(Ref. 2, p. 203)**

**6. (D)** The mandibular nerve passes through the foramen ovale. Each of the listed functions would be affected except the innervation of the stylohyoid muscle. The stylohyoid muscle is supplied by the facial nerve, which emerges from the skull through the stylomastoid foramen. **(Ref. 2, p. 265)**

**7. (A)** The glossopharyngeal nerve transmits general sensation and taste from the posterior one-third of the tongue. It also is sensory from most of the upper two-thirds of the pharynx and middle ear, and provides motor input to the stylopharyngeus muscle. **(Ref. 2, p. 239)**

**8. (E)** The facial artery winds around the inferior border of the mandible, anterior to the masseter muscle and deep to the overlying skin and platysma muscle. Its pulsations can be felt as it crosses the mandible. **(Ref. 2, p. 247)**

**9. (C)** The sympathetic trunk lies parallel and immediately deep to the carotid sheath in the neck. It is posterior to the carotid artery and ventral to the cervical muscles and transverse processes of the cervical vertebrae. The large superior ganglion is located at the level of the first cervical vertebra. **(Ref. 2, pp. 211–213)**

**10. (C)** The bony roof of the orbit is formed by the orbital plate of the frontal bone, and near the apex, by the lesser wing of the sphenoid bone. The frontal lobe of the brain lies on the orbital roof. **(Ref. 2, p. 291)**

**11. (D)** The promontory is the large bony eminence of the medial wall of the middle ear that is formed by the bulge of the basal turn of the cochlea. Superior to the promontory is the fenestra vestibuli and inferiorly is the fenestra cochlea. **(Ref. 2, p. 305)**

**12. (B)** The inferior alveolar artery is a branch of the first part of the maxillary artery in the infratemporal fossa. It enters the mandibular foramen with the nerve of the same name and supplies blood to the lower teeth and chin. (**Ref. 2,** p. 269)

13. (**B**)   The majority of the postganglionic sympathetic nerve fibers to the head have their cell bodies in the superior cervical chain ganglion. These fibers leave the chain ganglion and form the carotid plexus of nerves. (**Ref. 2,** p. 211)

14. (**C**)   The lateral cricoarytenoid muscle arises from the lateral surface of the arch of the cricoid cartilage. These fibers insert on the muscular process and function in drawing the process anteriorly, thus causing adduction of the vocal folds. (**Ref. 2,** p. 232)

15. (**E**)   The perpendicular (vertical) plate of the palatine bone forms the medial wall of the pterygopalatine fossa and separates this fossa from the nasal cavity. The roof is formed by the sphenoid bone, the posterior boundary is formed by the two pterygoid plates, and the maxilla is the anterior boundary. (**Ref. 2,** p. 265)

16. (**C**)   The middle meatus receives the drainage of the maxillary and anterior ethmoidal air cells via the hiatus semilunaris, the frontonasal duct, and the middle ethmoidal air cells via the bulla ethmoidalis. The nasolacrimal duct drains into the inferior meatus. (**Ref. 2,** pp. 281–283)

17. (**A**)   The submandibular gland receives its blood supply mainly from the facial artery as it courses deep to the gland. Venous drainage is via the facial vein, which courses superficial to the gland. (**Ref. 2,** p. 216)

18. (**C**)   The posterior superior alveolar nerve supplies the mucosa of the maxillary sinus, the maxillary molars, and the mucosa around the maxillary tuberosity. This nerve courses in the posterior wall of the maxillary sinus. (**Ref. 2,** p. 286)

19. (**D**)   The anterior two-thirds of the hard palate is formed by the palatine processes of the maxillae, and its posterior one-third is formed by the horizontal portions of the palatine bones. (**Ref. 2,** p. 277)

20. **(B)** The lingual nerve is sensory from the mucosa on the floor of the mouth and lingual gingiva. After receiving the chorda tympani, the lingual nerve conducts secretory fibers to the submandibular and sublingual glands and taste fibers from the anterior two-thirds of the tongue. The mandibular teeth are innervated by the inferior alveolar nerve. **(Ref. 2,** pp. 267–268)

21. **(B)** The sacculus is a membranous sac which, along with the utriculus, comprises part of the membranous labyrinth of the internal ear. Both of these lie in the bony vestibule and contain endolymph. **(Ref. 2,** p. 307)

22. **(D)** The mylohyoid nerve branches from the inferior alveolar nerve and courses in the mylohyoid groove to course with the submental artery. It innervates the mylohyoid and anterior belly of the digastric muscles. The mylohyoid nerve does not enter the mandibular foramen with the inferior alveolar nerve. **(Ref. 2,** pp. 267–268)

23. **(B)** The roots of the brachial plexus and the subclavian artery pass posterior to the anterior scalene muscle. The subclavian vein, suprascapular artery, and phrenic nerve pass anterior to the muscle. The thyrocervical trunk is medial to the muscle. **(Ref. 2,** pp. 221–225)

24. **(E)** Three muscles of mastication are involved in the elevation of the mandible. These are the masseter, medial pterygoid, and the anterior fibers of the temporalis. The posterior fibers of the temporalis retract the mandible. **(Ref. 2,** pp. 260–263)

25. **(D)** A lesion that compresses the neural contents with the jugular foramen would affect the ninth, tenth, and eleventh cranial nerves. The compression of the vagus cranial nerve might result in a loss of elevation of the soft palate. The other functions would not be possible. **(Ref. 2,** pp. 205–211)

26. **(E)** The ligature would stop the flow of blood to the maxillary artery, three of whose branches are the inferior alveolar, infraorbital, and middle meningeal arteries. It also would stop blood from flowing in the superficial temporal artery, one of the two terminal branches of the external carotid, the other being the maxil-

lary artery. The superior laryngeal artery is a branch of the superior thyroid artery and would not be involved in the occlusion. (**Ref. 2,** pp. 268–270)

27. **(D)** The palatine tonsil is embedded between palatine folds formed by the palatoglossus muscle anteriorly and the palatopharyngeus muscle posteriorly. In addition to its contact with these two muscles, the tonsil is in contact laterally with the superior pharyngeal constrictor and styloglossus muscles. (**Ref. 2,** pp. 280–281)

28. **(E)** The buccopharyngeal fascia surrounds the pharynx and esophagus. It thus extends from the skull to the posterior mediastinum and forms the anterior boundary of the retorpharyngeal space. A tonsillar abscess that invades the pharyngeal wall can extend into this space and reach the mediastinum. (**Ref. 2,** p. 226)

29. **(D)** The facial nerve exits the stylomastoid foramen and immediately innervates the posterior belly of the digastric and stylohyoid muscles. The facial nerve then courses through the parotid gland superficial to the retromandibular vein to innervate the muscles of facial expression. The submandibular and sublingual glands are innervated by fibers of the facial nerve carried in the chorda tympani. (**Ref. 2,** p. 252)

30. **(B)** The subclavian artery gives rise in part to the thyrocervical trunk and costocervical trunk. These supply each of the areas listed except for the floor of mouth, which receives its blood supply mainly from the lingual artery. (**Ref. 2,** pp. 221–225)

31. **(B)** The parotid gland receives secretomotor fibers from the glossopharyngeal nerve. The preganglionic fibers course within the tympanic and lesser petrosal nerves and synapse in the otic ganglion. The postganglionic fibers then course with the auriculotemporal nerve to reach the parotid gland. The nerve of the pterygoid canal conducts fibers of the facial nerve. (**Ref. 2,** pp. 251–253)

32. **(D)** The superficial layer of cervical fascia forms an outer cylindrical layer of fascia that encloses the trapezius and sternocleido-

mastoid muscles. It roofs the anterior and posterior cervical triangles. (Ref. 2, p. 191)

33. (E)  The preganglionic parasympathetic cell bodies of all parasympathetic pathways carried by cranial nerves III, VII, IX, and X are located in the brain. Postganglionic cell bodies are found in the autonomic terminal ganglia. (Ref. 2, p. 332)

34. (D)  The oculomotor nerve provides the parasympathetic innervation to the constrictor pupillae muscle. Damage to this nerve would result in a permanently dilated pupil, owing to the intact innervation of the dilator muscle of the pupil by sympathetic fibers. (Ref. 2, p. 295)

35. (B)  The ansa cervicalis provides innervation to most of the infrahyoid (strap) muscles. It is formed by superior and inferior roots. The latter are formed by the second and third cervical ventral rami of spinal nerves. (Ref. 2, p. 220)

36. (C)  The paired genioglossus muscles function in protrusion of the tongue and are innervated by the hypoglossal nerves. Following a lesion of the hypoglossal nerve, the tongue deviates to the side of the lesion when protruded. (Ref. 2, p. 275)

37. (E)  The palatine tonsils are in the oral part of the pharynx. The cricoid and arytenoid cartilages are deep to the mucosa and muscles of the laryngopharynx. The inferior pharyngeal constrictor is the main lateral and posterior muscular component of the lower pharynx, while the piriform recesses are the gutters located on each side of the inlet to the larynx. (Ref. 2, p. 236)

38. (E)  The deep petrosal nerve consists of postganglionic sympathetic nerve fibers whose cell bodies lie in the superior cervical sympathetic chain ganglion. These fibers are mostly vasomotor to the vessels of the nasal and palatine mucosae. (Ref. 2, p. 287)

39. (B)  The special visceral afferent fibers of the chorda tympani nerve, a branch of the facial nerve, convey impulses for taste from the anterior two-thirds of the tongue. They course partly with the lingual nerve and have their cell bodies in the geniculate ganglion. (Ref. 2, p. 309)

**40. (A)** The nasopalatine nerve, a branch of the maxillary nerve, conducts general somatic afferent fibers from the nasal septal mucosa and, by way of the incisive canal, from the anterior one-third of the hard palate. **(Ref. 2,** p. 285)

**41. (C)** The greater petrosal nerve, a branch of the facial nerve, contains preganglionic parasympathetic fibers that synapse in the pterygopalatine ganglion. The postganglionic fibers innervate mucus glands of the nose and palate, and the lacrimal gland. **(Ref. 2,** p. 287)

**42. (B)** The chorda tympani nerve, a branch of the facial nerve, contains, in addition to taste fibers, preganglionic parasympathetic nerve fibers that synapse in the submandibular ganglion. These fibers are secretomotor to the submandibular and sublingual glands. **(Ref. 2,** p. 216)

**43. (A)** The foramen ovale transmits the mandibular nerve and the accessory meningeal artery and vein. The mandibular nerve enters the infratemporal fossa, where it supplies the lower jaw, floor of the mouth, masticator muscles, and skin of the face. **(Ref. 2,** p. 265–270)

**44. (E)** The facial nerve and the eighth cranial nerve enter the skull through the internal acoustic meatus. This nerve courses through the facial canal, where it gives rise to the greater petrosal and chorda tympani nerves, and exits the skull at the stylomastoid foramen. **(Ref. 2,** p. 309)

**45. (B)** The foramen rotundum transmits the maxillary nerve. The maxillary nerve courses through the pteryopalatine fossa, where it supplies the area of the maxilla. **(Ref. 2,** p. 285)

**46. (C)** The chorda tympani nerve leaves the middle ear through the petrotympanic fissure to enter the infratemporal fossa. It then joins the lingual nerve, where its neurons are visceral motor to the submandibular and sublingual glands and transmit taste from the anterior two-thirds of the tongue. **(Ref. 2,** p. 310)

**47. (D)** The ophthalmic nerve leaves the cranial cavity to enter the orbit by passing through the superior orbital fissure. In the orbit, it divides into the frontal, lacrimal, and nasociliary nerves to supply the tissues of the orbit. (Ref 2, p. 297)

48. **(A)** The piriform recesses are the gutters located on either side of the laryngeal inlet. The mucous membrane receives sensory innervation from the internal branch of the superior laryngeal nerve. **(Ref. 2,** p. 236)

49. **(C)** The stylopharyngeus muscle is one of the three vertical muscles that elevate the pharynx during swallowing. This muscle is innervated by the glossopharyngeal nerve. **(Ref. 2,** p. 238)

50. **(B)** The external branch of the superior laryngeal nerve innervates the cricothyroid muscle, which functions in increasing tension on the vocal folds. The external branch of the nerve courses with the superior thyroid artery. **(Ref. 2,** p. 234)

51. **(D)** The inferior laryngeal nerve is the superior continuation of the recurrent laryngeal nerve. The inferior nerve innervates the muscles of the larynx except the cricothyroid, and conveys sensory fibers from the mucosa of the lower part of the laryngeal cavity. **(Ref. 2,** p. 234)

52. **(B)** The infraorbital nerve courses across the roof of the maxillary sinus in the infraorbital groove. In this position, the nerve could be damaged by a fracture of the maxillary sinus. **(Ref. 2,** p. 286)

53. **(C)** The mental nerve is the terminal end of the inferior alveolar nerve. The fibers in this nerve pass through the foramen ovale and mandibular foramen before exiting the mental foramen. **(Ref. 2,** p. 268)

54. **(F)** The great auricular nerve is one of the cutaneous nerves that derives from contributions from the second and third cervical spinal nerves. The transverse cervical and lesser occipital cutaneous nerves derive from these same nerves. **(Ref. 2,** p. 191)

55. **(D)** The buccal nerve is a branch of the mandibular nerve. It is sensory from the buccal nucosa of the cheek, from the skin over-

lying the buccinator muscle, and from the buccal gingiva. (**Ref. 2,** p. 267)

56. **(H)**  The auriculotemporal nerve branches from the mandibular nerve high in the infratemporal fossa. This nerve encircles the middle meningeal artery and passes inferior to the zygomatic arch to reach skin of the face and temporal area. (**Ref. 2,** p. 267)

57. **(C)**  The inferior pharyngeal constrictor muscle is one of the three circular muscles of the pharynx. The muscle is attached to the thyroid and cricoid cartilages and is innervated by the pharyngeal branches of the vagus nerve. (**Ref. 2,** p. 237)

58. **(A)**  The thyrohyoid muscle is one of the infrahyoid (strap) muscles. It is innervated by motor fibers derived from the first cervical spinal nerve, which join and course with the hypoglossal nerve. These fibers leave the hypoglossal nerve in the carotid triangle to enter the muscle. (**Ref. 2.** p. 197)

59. **(F)**  The genioglossus muscle originates from the mental spine with a small attachment to the hyoid bone. These fibers curve into the tongue, forming the major bulk of the tongue. The genioglossus muscle protracts the tongue and is innervated by the hypoglossal nerve. (**Ref. 2,** p. 275)

60. **(B)**  The esophagus receives its motor and sensory innervation from the recurrent laryngeal nerve as it ascends the neck between the trachea and esophagus. The nerve also supplies the trachea. (**Ref. 2,** p. 241)

# THE UPPER EXTREMITY

61. **(E)**  The posterior circumflex humeral artery, a branch of the third part of the axillary artery, accompanies the axillary nerve through the quadrangular space. The artery contributes to the collateral blood supply around the shoulder. The artery and nerve are often damaged by a fracture of the surgical neck of the humerus. (**Ref. 2,** p. 118)

62. **(D)** Flexion of the arm at the shoulder is performed by the biceps brachii, corocobrachialis, and pectoralis major muscles. The other muscles listed function in the movements of the scapula or abduction of the arm. (**Ref. 2**, pp. 171–174)

63. **(D)** Because the radial nerve spirals around the humerus in the radial groove, it is more likely than other nerves in the arm to be injured in fractures of the middle of the humerus. The deep brachial artery runs with the nerve. (**Ref. 2**, pp. 130–132)

64. **(E)** The latissimus dorsi muscle covers the lower half of the posterior thoracic region and the lumbar region. Its action is to extend, adduct, and medially rotate the arm. It is innervated by the thoracodorsal nerve. (**Ref. 2**, p. 92)

65. **(B)** Three muscles insert on the greater tubercle of the humerus. These are the supraspinatus, infraspinatus, and teres minor. The loss of these muscles from injury would affect abduction and lateral rotation of the humerus. (**Ref. 2**, pp. 95–96)

66. **(D)** The boundaries of the axilla are formed by the pectoralis major and minor muscles anteriorly; posteriorly by the latissimus dorsi, teres major, and subscapularis muscles; medially by the serratus anterior muscle; and laterally by the coracobrachialis and biceps brachii muscles. (**Ref. 2**, p. 114)

67. **(C)** The median nerve is formed by contributions from the lateral and medial cords of the brachial plexus. It crosses the ventral surface of the axillary artery and travels in the neurovascular compartment of the arm. The median nerve innervates muscles only in the forearm and hand. (**Ref. 2**, pp. 129–130)

68. **(A)** The distal end of the spinal cord tapers to form the conus medullaris, which terminates at the level of the second lumbar vertebra. The transverse level of the iliac crest is at the fourth lumbar vertebra, which would insure that the needle does not injure the spinal cord. (**Ref. 2**, p. 353)

69. **(B)** The superficial palmar arterial arch is located in the central compartment of the palm and is formed mainly by the superficial branch of the ulnar artery. It is distal to the position of the deep

palmar arch and superficial to the long flexor tendons of the palm. (**Ref. 2,** p. 161)

70. **(E)** In the forearm, the ulnar nerve innervates the flexor carpi ulnaris and ulnar half of the flexor digitorum profundus muscles. This latter muscle flexes the distal phalanx of the fourth and fifth digits and the wrist. (**Ref. 2,** pp. 146–148)

71. **(B)** The two primary lateral rotators of the humerus are the teres minor and infraspinatus muscles. The former is innervated by the axillary nerve and the latter by the suprascapular nerve. Both the teres minor and infraspinatus insert on the greater tubercle of the humerus. (**Ref. 2,** pp. 95–96)

72. **(B)** The erector spinae is the largest muscle of the deep, intrinsic muscles of the back. This group of muscles is innervated segmentally by the dorsal rami of spinal nerves, and functions in movements of the trunk. (**Ref. 2,** p. 336)

73. **(E)** Injury to the median nerve in the middle of the arm would affect the pronator teres, pronator quadratus, flexor carpi radialis, opponens pollicis, abductor pollicis brevis, lateral two lumbicals, flexor digitorum superficial, radial half of the flexor digitorum profundus, and flexor pollicis brevis muscles. (**Ref. 2,** pp. 145–146)

74. **(D)** The radial artery runs through the anatomic snuffbox, the region bounded by the tendons of the extensor pollicis longus and brevis muscles on the dorsum of the thumb. The scaphoid bone could also be damaged. (**Ref. 2,** pp. 154–155)

75. **(A)** Ligation of the brachial artery in the distal third of the arm would still permit blood to reach the forearm by means of the radial collateral and middle collateral branches of the deep brachial and superior ulnar collateral arteries. The ulnar artery would be distal to ligation and not provide any collateral blood flow. (**Ref. 2,** pp. 148–150)

76. **(B)** The deep branch of the ulnar nerve branches from the ulnar nerve at the base of the hypothenar eminence of the hand. It penetrates and innervates the hypothenar muscles as well as the dorsal

and palmar interossei. The palmaris longus muscle is innervated by the median nerve. (**Ref. 2,** p. 167)

**77. (E)** The medial pectoral nerve is a branch of the medial cord. All the other nerves listed, plus the lower subscapular nerve, might be affected by an injury to the posterior cord of the brachial plexus. (**Ref. 2,** pp. 121–122)

**78. (B)** Owing to the loss of the adductor pollicis muscle resulting from the injury, the thumb would be abducted by the intact long and short abductor muscles of the thumb, which are innervated by the radial and median nerves, respectively. (**Ref. 2,** pp. 168–169)

**79. (B)** The superficial radial nerve branches from the radial nerve in the cubital fossa and becomes a cutaneous nerve that descends the forearm deep to the brachioradialis muscle. The superficial radial nerve is sensory from the dorsal surface of the thumb. (**Ref. 2,** p. 147)

**80. (E)** Distal to the carpal tunnel, the median nerve (motor branch) innervates the three muscles of thenar compartment (opponens pollicis, flexor pollicis brevis, and abductor pollicis brevis) and the first two lumbrical muscles. Cutaneous branches of the nerve are also sensory from the palmar surface of the lateral three digits and the lateral side of the fourth digit. (**Ref. 2,** p. 163)

**81. (D)** The eighth cervical spinal nerve provides segmental cutaneous innervation to the ulnar side of the forearm and hand. The cephalic aspect of the limb is supplied by cutaneous fibers of the 5th cervical nerve. (**Ref. 2,** p. 122)

**82. (A)** Damage to the median nerve in the arm would affect flexion and abduction of the wrist, flexion of the thumb, and pronation of the forearm. Supination is a function of muscles supplied by the musculocutaneous and deep branch of the radial nerve. (**Ref. 2,** p. 145)

**83. (C)** Adduction of the second, fourth, and fifth digits is a function of the palmar interossei muscles, which are innervated by branches of the ulnar nerve. These muscles also assist in interphalangeal extension of the digits. (**Ref. 2,** p. 168)

**84. (C)** The radial artery does not enter the central compartment of the palm, but courses dorsally through the anatomic snuffbox to the dorsum of the hand. There it pierces the first dorsal interossous muscle to form the deep palmar arterial arch. (**Ref. 2,** p. 154)

**85. (D)** The medial cord of the brachial plexus is formed by the anterior division fibers of C-8 and T-1 spinal cord segments. It is medial to the axillary artery and contributes to the median, ulnar, medial pectoral, and cutaneous nerves. (**Ref. 2,** pp. 119–123)

**86. (C)** The dorsal roots of spinal nerves convey only sensory fibers and do not carry any sympathetic motor fibers. The dorsal root ganglia are located on the dorsal roots at the intervertebral foramina, where they contain sensory cell bodies. (**Ref. 2,** pp. 35–36)

**87. (B)** The cephalic vein begins from the lateral side of the dorsal venous arch of the hand. The vein ascends in the superficial fascia on the lateral aspect of the forearm and arm. In the deltopectoral triangle, the cephalic vein pierces the deep fascia to drain into the axillary vein. (**Ref. 2,** p. 101)

**88. (B)** All of the structures listed except the ulnar artery course through the carpal tunnel deep to the flexor retinaculum. The ulnar vessels and nerve cross superficial to the retinaculum to enter the palm. (**Ref. 2,** pp. 152–154)

**89. (E)** The superior ulnar collateral artery arises from the brachial artery near the middle of the arm and accompanies the ulnar nerve. The artery and nerve course posterior to the medial epicondyle to enter the forearm, where the artery contributes to the collateral blood supply at the elbow. (**Ref 2,** p. 133)

**90. (B)** The common interosseous artery, usually the largest branch of the ulnar artery in the forearm, gives rise to the anterior and posterior interosseous arteries. These two arteries supply the deep tissues of the flexor and extensor surfaces of the forearm. (**Ref. 2,** p. 149)

**91. (B)** The ulnar artery, after if branches from the brachial artery, accompanies the ulnar nerve in the middle of the forearm deep to the flexor carpi ulnaris muscle. Both the artery and the nerve enter the hand superficial to the flexor retinaculum. (**Ref. 2,** p. 150)

**92. (A)** The radial artery passes diagonally onto the back of the hand and contributes laterally to the dorsal carpal arterial arch before penetrating the first dorsal interosseous muscle. (**Ref. 2,** p. 154)

**93. (B)** The flexor digitorum superficialis muscle is innervated by the median nerve as the nerve courses deep to the muscle in the center of the forearm. This muscle flexes the wrist and digits two through five. (**Ref. 2,** p. 141)

**94. (E)** The abductor pollicis brevis muscle is in the thenar compartment of the hand and is innervated by the motor branch of the median nerve. This recurrent branch of the median nerve occurs just distal to the flexor retinaculum. (**Ref. 2,** p. 159)

**95. (A)** The brachioradialis muscle is the most superficial muscle on the radial side of the forearm. It is innervated by the radial nerve at the lateral aspect of the arm, before the radial nerve divides into the superficial and deep radial nerves. (**Ref. 2,** p. 136)

**96. (E)** The opponens pollicis muscle is supplied by the motor branch of the median nerve. The action of the opponens pollicis is to allow opposition of the thumb to the other digits. (**Ref. 2,** p. 161)

**97. (A)** The triceps brachii muscle receives its innervation from the radial nerve. There are several radial nerve branches to the muscle, either proximal to or in the radial groove on the posterior surface of the humerus. (**Ref. 2,** p. 126)

**98. (A)** The long thoracic nerve is formed by nerve fibers of C-5, C-6, and C-7, and innervates the serratus anterior muscle. Loss of this muscle results in a flaring out of the scapula from the back (winged scapula). (**Ref. 2,** p. 120)

**99. (E)** The median and ulnar nerves derive from the brachial plexus and course through the arm, but do not innervate any muscles of the arm. They innervate the preaxial muscles of the forearm and hand, the median nerve primarily to the forearm, and the ulnar nerve primarily to the hand. (**Ref. 2,** pp. 129–130)

100. **(J)**   The suprascapular nerve is a branch of the superior trunk, and courses across the shoulder to pass deep to the superior transverse scapular ligament. This nerve innervates the supraspinatus and infraspinatus muscles. (**Ref. 2,** p. 120)

101. **(D)**   The radial nerve is a branch of the posterior cord and innervates the extensor muscles on the posterior aspect of the forearm. These muscles function in extension of the wrist and their loss of function would cause wrist drop. (**Ref. 2,** p. 147)

# THE LOWER EXTREMITY

102. **(D)**   The fibular artery is the largest branch of the posterior tibial artery and is an important muscular artery on the fibular side of the leg. It serves as a collateral vessel between the posterior and anterior tibial arteries. (**Ref. 2,** p. 620)

103. **(B)**   When the common fibular nerve is paralyzed, there is foot drop due to loss of the extensors of the foot, and a turning in of the foot (loss of eversion) due to paralysis of the fibular muscles. (**Ref. 2,** p. 621)

104. **(E)**   As the deep fibular nerve curves around the neck of the fibula and enters the anterior compartment of the leg, it is joined on its medial side by the anterior tibial artery. (**Ref. 2,** p. 618)

105. **(B)**   The tibial collateral ligament is a strong, flat band that extends form the tubercle of the medial femoral condyle to the medial condyle of the tibia and the medial aspect of its shaft. The deeper fibers of the tibial collateral ligament attach to the medial meniscus. (**Ref. 2,** p. 637)

106. **(A)**   The gluteus maximus muscle is a powerful extensor of the thigh and a strong extensor of the trunk. It aids in holding the knee in extension during standing. It also is a strong lateral rotator, and the inferior gluteal nerve innervates it. (**Ref. 2,** p. 588)

**107. (A)** Paralysis of the tibial nerve results in loss of muscles of the posterior compartment of the leg and sole of the foot. Plantar flexion of the ankle is lost; the toes cannot be flexed. Sensory loss also occurs on the sole of the foot. (**Ref. 2**, p. 621)

**108. (B)** The deep femoral artery, the largest branch of the femoral artery, gives rise to perforating arteries, which are the primary blood supply to the muscles in the posterior compartment of the thigh. (**Ref. 2**, p. 601)

**109. (A)** The medial femoral muscles are all preaxial adductors of the thigh and are supplied by the obturator nerve. The gluteus medius muscle is a strong abductor of the thigh. (**Ref. 2,** p. 593)

**110. (C)** The sartorius muscle inserts into the medial surface of the upper tibia. Its contraction produces flexion, abduction, and lateral rotation of the thigh. The sartorius forms the lateral border of the femoral triangle and is innervated by the femoral nerve. (**Ref. 2,** p. 590)

**111. (C)** The lateral rotators of the thigh are the gluteus maximus, piriformis, quadratus femoris, obturator internus, superior and inferior gemelli, and obturator externus muscles. The gluteus minimus muscle is an abductor and medial rotator of the thigh. (**Ref. 2,** p. 634)

**112. (C)** The lesser sciatic foramen is bounded anteriorly by the tuberosity and body of the ischium, superiorly by the spine of the ischium and sacrospinous ligament, and posteriorly by the sacrotuberous ligament. Passing through this notch are the obturator internus muscle and its nerve and the internal pudendal vessels and nerve. (**Ref. 2,** p. 568)

**113. (E)** The femoral sheath is derived from the transversalis fascia and encloses the proximal portions of the femoral vessels. The femoral nerve lies lateral to the sheath, while the inguinal ligament is anterior to it. The sheath is divided into three compartments, a lateral one containing the femoral artery, a middle one for the femoral vein, and a medial one for some deep inguinal lymph nodes. (**Ref. 2,** p. 586)

**114. (C)** The adductor canal contains the femoral artery and vein, the saphenous nerve, and the nerve to the vastus medialis muscle. The deep femoral artery is posterior to the canal. (**Ref. 2,** p. 586)

**115. (C)** The biceps femoris muscle is a flexor of the leg. After the leg is flexed, the muscle can rotate the tibia laterally on the femur. The long head of the biceps also extends the thigh. The biceps femoris has a double innervation, with one component coming from the tibial portion of the sciatic nerve to the long head and the other consisting of a branch of the common peroneal division of the sciatic nerve to the short head of the muscle. (**Ref. 2,** p. 596)

**116. (C)** Both the tibialis anterior and the deep posterior leg muscles have powerful actions in inversion of the foot. In addition, the tibialis anterior has a strong action on dorsiflexion of the foot, while the tibialis posterior is a powerful plantar flexor of the foot. (**Ref. 2,** pp. 610–614)

**117. (A)** The sartorius muscle is innervated by the femoral nerve. All of the other muscles listed, plus the adductor brevis, are innervated by the obturator nerve. The obturator nerve passes through the obturator canal from the pelvis to enter the medial compartment of the thigh. (**Ref. 2,** pp. 590–593)

**118. (E)** The posterior compartment of the leg contains all of the structures listed except the medial plantar artery. This artery is a branch of the posterior tibial artery in the sole of the foot. (**Ref. 2,** pp. 613–619)

**119. (A)** The dorsalis pedis artery is the continuation of the anterior tibial artery, which is found on the dorsum of the foot. All other arteries would be affected by ligation of the posterior tibial artery. (**Ref. 2,** p. 618)

**120. (E)** The extensor hallucis longus muscle is innervated by the deep fibular nerve. The tibial nerve supplies the gastrocnemius, plantaris, soleus, popliteus, tibialis posterior, flexor digitorum longus, and flexor hallucis longus muscles on the posterior leg. (**Ref. 2,** p. 610)

**121. (E)** Cutaneous loss would involve most of the heel and sole, owing to the loss of the tibial nerve, whose branches, the medial calcaneal and medial and lateral plantar nerves, supply the greater part of these two regions. **(Ref. 2, p. 583)**

**122. (A)** The thickened lateral portion of the fascia lata is named the iliotibial tract. The tract receives the tendinous insertion of the tensor fasciae latae and gluteus maximus muscles. The iliotibial tract helps stabaliize the lower limb during standing. **(Ref. 2, p. 584)**

**123. (C)** The inferior gluteal nerve is a postaxial branch from the sacral plexus, with fibers derived from L-5, S-1, and S-2. It supplies only the gluteus maximus muscle, and is therefore important in movements of extension and lateral rotation of the hip. **(Ref. 2, p. 589)**

**124. (C)** The base of the femoral triangle is formed by the inguinal ligament. Its sides are the sartorius muscle laterally and the adductor longus muscle medially. The femoral vessels and nerve occupy the triangle. Distally the apex of the triangle continues into the adductor canal. **(Ref. 2, p. 585)**

**125. (C)** The superficial muscles of the posterior leg are the gastrocnemius, soleus, and plantaris. The combined tendons of these muscles form the calcaneal (Achilles) tendon, which inserts on the calcaneus. The muscles are innervated by the tibial nerve and are plantar flexors of the foot. **(Ref. 2, p. 612)**

**126. (D)** The lateral intermuscular septum of the thigh extends from the iliotibial tract to the lateral margin of the linea aspera on the dorsum of the femur. The septum separates the biceps femoris muscle in the posterior compartment from the vastus lateralis muscle in the anterior compartment. **(Ref. 2, p. 585)**

**127. (C)** Only one muscle originates from the anterior inferior iliac spine, the rectus femoris. The sartorius and tensor fasciae latae muscles originate from the anterior superior iliac spine. **(Ref. 2, p. 591)**

**128. (A)** The quadratus plantae muscle is innervated by the lateral plantar nerve. The other muscles receive innervation from the medial plantar nerve after branching from the tibial nerve deep to the flexor retinaculum. The medial plantar nerve courses in the big-toe compartment of the foot. (**Ref. 2,** p. 632)

**129. (D)** The sartorius muscle crosses the thigh obliquely and forms the roof of the adductor canal. The vastus medialis muscle is the lateral boundary of the canal and the adductor longus and magnus muscles form the medial boundary. (**Ref. 2,** p. 586)

**130. (C)** The adductor hiatus is formed by a splitting of the inferior fibers of the adductor magnus muscle. The femoral vessels pass through this opening to enter the popliteal fossa on the dorsum of the knee. There they are named the popliteal artery and vein. (**Ref. 2,** p. 595)

**131. (D)** The plantar arterial arch is formed laterally from the lateral plantar artery where it goes deep into the interosseous compartment. Medially, the arch is completed by the deep plantar artery, a branch of the dorsalis pedis artery. (**Ref. 2,** p. 631)

**132. (E)** The main support of the ankle joint is provided by the distal end of the tibia and the trochlea of the talus. These two bones bear most of the weight on the foot and are the ones most often broken. (**Ref. 2,** p. 642)

**133. (A)** Extension of the knee is the primary function of the quadriceps femoris muscle. This muscle is divided into four parts: vastus lateralis, vastus intermedius, vastus medialis, and rectus femoris muscles. These are innervated by the femoral nerve and are located in the anterior compartment of the thigh. (**Ref. 2,** p. 591)

**134. (C)** The femoral nerve is lateral to the femoral artery. The motor branches of the femoral nerve are distributed to muscles in the anterior compartment of the thigh. Below the knee, there are only cutaneous branches from the femoral nerve to the medial side of the leg. (**Ref. 2,** p. 606)

**135. (B)** The popliteal fossa is the diamond-shaped area posterior to the knee. Superiorly, the lateral boundary of the fossa is formed by the biceps femoris muscle and medially by the semitendinosus and semimembranosus muscles. (**Ref. 2,** p. 586)

**136. (E)** The lateral plantar nerve is similar to the ulnar nerve of the hand, and innervates most of the muscles of the foot. It branches from the tibial nerve deep to the flexor digitorum, and courses deep to the quadratus plantae muscle to reach the lateral side of the foot. (**Ref. 2,** p. 630)

**137. (B)** The rectus femoris muscle is in the anterior thigh and is an extensor of the leg. The other muscles function in flexion of the leg at the knee. (**Ref. 2,** p. 591)

**138. (C)** The quadratus femoris muscle inserts on the intertrochanteric crest of the femur. It serves as a strong lateral rotator. (**Ref. 2,** p. 591)

**139. (A)** The iliopsoas muscle courses in the anterior compartment of the thigh and inserts on the lesser trochanter, where it is a strong flexor of the thigh. (**Ref. 2,** p. 513)

**140. (B)** The gluteus medius muscle originates from the posterior surface of the ileum and inserts on the lateral and posterior surfaces of the greater trochanter. The gluteus medius and minimus muscles are important in locking the pelvis during walking. (**Ref. 2,** pp. 588–589)

# THE THORAX

**141. (E)** The superior mediastinum is bounded superiorly by the first rib, inferiorly by a horizontal plane through the sternal angle, and laterally by the mediastinal (parietal) pleura. (**Ref. 2,** p. 370)

**142. (B)** The major portion of the sternocostal surface of the heart is occupied by the right ventricle, with additional contributions from the right atrium and left ventricle. (**Ref. 2,** p. 378)

**143. (B)** The right vagus nerve crosses the first part of the subclavian artery, continues its descent alongside the trachea, and passes dorsal to the root of the right lung. (**Ref. 2,** p. 386)

**144. (C)** The coronary sinus receives the great cardiac vein, middle cardiac vein, small cardiac vein, posterior vein of the left ventricle, and oblique vein of the left atrium. The anterior cardiac vein drains a portion of the right ventricle and empties directly into the right atrium. **(Ref. 2, p. 388)**

**145. (B)** The phrenic nerve is found in the middle and superior mediastina. The posterior mediastinum contains the thoracic aorta, azygos and hemizygous veins, vagus and splanchnic nerves, tracheal bifurcation, esophagus, and thoracic duct. **(Ref. 2, p. 386)**

**146. (C)** The external jugular vein drains into the subclavain vein. The brachiocephalic veins are formed by the internal jugular and subclavian veins and receive the vertebral, internal thoracic, inferior thyroid, and posterior intercostal veins. **(Ref. 2, p. 384)**

**147. (C)** The bicuspid valve is in the left ventricle. Related to the chamber of the right ventricle are the right atrioventricular orifice, tricuspid valve, chordae tendineae, trabeculae carneae, supraventricular crest, papillary muscles, and interventricular septum. **(Ref. 2, p. 393)**

**148. (B)** The greater splanchnic nerve is derived from the T-5 to T-9 thoracic spinal nerve. The least splanchnic nerve is formed by T-12 and the lesser splanchnic nerve by T-10 and T-11. **(Ref. 2, p. 416)**

**149. (C)** The left coronary artery divides between the pulmonary trunk and the left auricle into the circumflex and anterior interventricular arteries. These two arteries supply the major parts of the left ventricle, left atrium, and interventricular septum, and parts of the right ventricle. **(Ref. 2, p. 387)**

**150. (D)** Referred pain during a heart attack is usually conveyed by the second thoracic spinal nerve via the left intercostobrachial nerve. The latter communicates on the medial aspect of the arm with the medial brachial cutaneous nerve. **(Ref. 2, p. 103)**

**151. (D)** The coronary sulcus separates the two ventricles from the two atria and contains the right coronary artery, circumflex artery, great cardiac vein, and coronary sinus. The middle cardiac vein is located in the posterior interventricular sulcus. (**Ref. 2,** p. 380)

**152.** (**B**) The brachiocephalic veins are posterior to the sternum and are therefore the most anterior of the structures in the superior mediastinum. Deep to the veins are the major arterial branches and the vagus and phrenic nerves. (**Ref. 2,** p. 384)

**153.** (**D**) The left subclavian artery is a branch of the aortic arch in the superior mediastinum. The other vessels are branches of the descending aorta in the posterior mediastinum, and supply the parietal and visceral structures of the thorax. (**Ref. 2,** p. 384)

**154.** (**A**) The greater, lesser, and least splanchnic nerves are preganglionic sympathetic fibers that course through the diaphragm to synapse in collateral ganglia in the abdomen. These nerves also contain visceral afferent nerve fibers. (**Ref. 2,** p. 416)

**155.** (**B**) The white rami communicantes are found only in spinal nerves T-1 to L-2 and conduct preganglionic sympathetic fibers. The other characteristics listed are typical for all spinal nerves. (**Ref. 2,** p. 36)

**156.** (**C**) The trachea is anterior to the esophagus in the superior mediastinum. The vertebral column is posterior to the esophagus. The aortic arch courses on the left side of the esophagus and trachea. (**Ref. 2,** p. 399)

**157.** (**E**) The thoracic duct is the largest lymphatic channel. It begins in the abdomen at the cisterna chyli and ascends through the thorax. The thoracic duct crosses to the right side of the vertebral column by coursing posterior to the esophagus in the superior mediastinum and terminates in the root of the neck. (**Ref. 2,** p. 412)

**158.** (**D**) The posterior interventricular sulcus separates the left ventricle from the right ventricle. It is located on the diaphragmatic surface of the heart and contains the posterior interventricular artery and middle cardiac vein. (**Ref. 2,** p. 380)

**159.** (**E**) The parietal pleura lines the thoracic cavity and is divided into diaphragmatic, cervical, costal, and mediastinal parts. It is the outer boundary of the pleural cavity and is fused to the inner surface of the chest wall. (**Ref. 2**, p. 371)

**160.** **(D)**  Septal arteries arise from the anterior and posterior interventricular arteries, which penetrate into the septum. Those septal arteries that arise from the anterior interventricular artery supply the anterior two-thirds of the interventricular septum, while those arising from the posterior interventricular artery supply the posterior one-third of the septum. (**Ref. 2**, p. 387)

**161.** **(A)**  The esophagus passes posterior to the bifurcation of the trachea and enters the posterior mediastinum. It deviates to the left where it is located posterior to the left atrium. The pericardium separates the atrium and esophagus. (**Ref. 2**, pp. 408–409)

**162.** **(C)**  The costodiaphragmatic recess is the inferior part of the pleural cavity in the midaxillary line, deep to the 8th and 9th intercostal spaces. It is not part of the thoracic cavity, and contains small amount of serous fluid. (**Ref. 2**, p. 371)

**163.** **(A)**  At the root of the left lung, the left pulmonary artery is located superior to the bronchus. On the right, the pulmonary artery is ventral to the bronchus. The pulmonary veins are ventral to the bronchus on both sides. (**Ref. 2**, p. 406)

**164.** **(A)**  The horizontal fissure is found only in the right lung and separates the superior and middle lobes of the lung. The oblique fissure is common to both the right and left lungs. (**Ref. 2**, p. 404)

**165.** **(E)**  The bachiocephalic trunk bifurcates deep to the right sternoclavicular joint, which is at the level of the first rib. Each of the other landmarks occurs at the plane of the sternal angle formed by the articulation of the second rib and the sternum. (**Ref. 2**, p. 383)

**166.** **(C)**  The tubercle of the rib is a posterior projection at the junction of the neck and shaft of a rib. It articulates with the transverse process of a vertebra. Movements at this articulation occur during respiration. (**Ref. 2**, p. 360)

**167.** **(A)**  The superior vena cava originates deep to the right first costal cartilage from the union of the right and left brachiocephalic veins. The superior vena cava enters the right artium at the level of the third right costal cartilage. (**Ref. 2,** p. 384)

**168.** **(E)** The right atrium begins deep to the third rib. It constitutes the right border of the heart and extends inferiorly to a point deep to the right sixth costal cartilage. (**Ref. 2,** p. 378)

**169.** **(A)** The great cardiac vein begins at the apex of the heart and ascends in the anterior interventricular sulcus and coronary sulcus to empty into the left extremity of the coronary sinus. It receives venous flow from the right and left ventricles and left atrium. (**Ref. 2,** p. 388)

**170.** **(E)** The coronary sinus is located in the posterior part of the coronary sulcus between the left atrium and left ventricle. It empties into the right atrium after receiving most of the venous flow from the cardiac musculature. (**Ref. 2,** p. 388)

**171.** **(D)** The middle cardiac vein begins at the apex of the heart, ascends in the posterior interventricular sulcus, and empties into the coronary sinus. It drains the diaphragmatic aspect of both ventricles. (**Ref. 2,** p. 388)

**172.** **(C)** The small cardiac vein begins along the acute margin of the heart. It turns posteriorly in the coronary sulcus and terminates in the right end of the coronary sinus. It accompanies the right coronary artery. (**Ref. 2,** p. 389)

**173.** **(A)** The ascending aorta appears in the radiograph along the right border of the sternum. The ascending aorta begins at the base of the heart at the level of the third costal cartilage and ascends to the sternal angle, where it becomes the arch of the aorta. The two branches of the ascending aorta are the right and left coronary arteries. (**Ref. 2,** p. 381)

**174.** **(B)** The left ventricle forms most of the left border of the heart, lying deep to the third to fifth ribs on the left chest wall. The left ventricle often shows the greatest increase in size following chronic enlargement of the heart. (**Ref. 2,** p. 378)

**175. (C)**   The apex of the heart is the far left point of the heart, and is formed by the junction of the left border and left end of the diaphragmatic surface of the heart. The apex is located deep to the fifth intercostal space, about 9 cm from the left border of the sternum. **(Ref. 2, p. 378)**

**176. (D)**   The superior surface of the diaphragm is easily identified by the contrast between the diaphragmatic muscle and the darkness of the air in the thorax. The diaphragmatic surface of the heart rests on the diaphragm, and the fibrous pericardium is firmly attached to the superior diaphragmatic surface. **(Ref. 2, p. 375)**

**177. (E)**   the right border of the heart is formed almost exclusively by the right aspect of the right atrium. This border descends from deep to the third costal cartilage to the sixth costal cartilage. **(Ref. 2, p. 379)**

**178. (I)**   The posterior interventricular artery is the descending, terminal end of the right coronary artery. It courses in the posterior interventricular sulcus with the middle cardiac vein, and supplies parts of the left and right ventricles. **(Ref. 2, p. 387)**

**179. (K)**   The right coronary artery branches from the ascending aorta between the right atrium and the infundibulum of the right ventricle. The artery descends in the coronary sulcus, supplying the anterior surfaces of the right atrium and right ventricle, and then turns around the right border of the heart, where it continues as the posterior interventricular artery on the diaphragmatic surface of the heart. The right coronary artery gives rise to the important sinuatrial and atrioventricular nodal arteries. **(Ref. 2, p. 387)**

**180. (E)**   The circumflex artery arises from the bifurcation of the left coronary artery and courses between the left auricle and left ventricle. The circumflex artery passes around the left border of the heart in the coronary sulcus, deep to the great cardiac vein and coronary sinus. It supplies parts of the left ventricle and left atrium. **(Ref. 2, p. 387)**

**181. (A)**   The superior vena cava begins deep to the first costal cartilage, from the confluence of the right and left brachiocephalic veins. It descends along the right border of the sternum and drains into the right atrium at the base of the heart at the level of the third costal cartilage. (**Ref. 2,** p. 384)

**182.** **(F)** The anterior interventricular artery is one of the two major branches of the left coronary artery. It descends in the anterior interventricular sulcus with the great cardiac vein and supplies parts of the right and left ventricles and the interventricular septum. (**Ref. 2,** p. 387)

**183.** **(C)** The pulmonary trunk is the superior continuation of the infundibulum of the right ventricle. The flow of blood from the right ventricle is controlled by the pulmonary semilunar valves. The pulmonary trunk divides into the right and left pulmonary arteries at the level of the sternal angle to carry blood to the two lungs. (**Ref. 2,** p. 386)

**184.** **(B)** The aortic arch begins and terminates at the level of the sternal angle. The arch of the aorta courses to the left and posteriorly over the bifurcation of the pulmonary trunk to reach the left side of the vertebral column. The three branches of the aortic arch are the brachiocephalic trunk, left common carotid artery, and left subclavian artery. (**Ref. 2,** p. 383)

**185.** **(L)** The sinuatrial nodal artery is the first branch from the right side of the right coronary artery. The sinuatrial artery courses posterior to an encircles the superior vena cava to reach the superior end of the terminal sulcus, where the sinuatrial node is embedded. (**Ref. 2,** p. 387)

# THE ABDOMEN, PERINEUM, AND PELVIS

**186.** **(E)** Fibers of the internal abdominal oblique muscle, together with those of the transverse abdominis, form the falx inguinalis. The other structures are derived from the external abdominal oblique muscle and fascia. (**Ref. 2,** p. 425)

**187.** **(C)** The parasympathetic preganglionic nerve fibers to the wall of the urinary bladder have their cell bodies in the second, third, and fourth sacral spinal cord segments and are carried in the pelvic splanchnic nerves. (**Ref. 2,** p. 540)

**188. (B)** If the inferior mesenteric vein was ligated, blood could still return to the hepatic portal vein by means of anastomoses between the left and middle colic veins, which are tributaries to the marginal vein. (**Ref. 2,** pp. 469–470)

**189. (C)** The venous drainage of the digestive tract is to the liver by way of the hepatic portal vein. Metastases in these organs would first appear in the liver. The kidney drains directly via the renal vein into the inferior vena cava, and metastases would therefore travel through the right atrium and ventricle and into the pulmonary artery to the lung. (**Ref. 2,** pp. 487–489)

**190. (E)** The inguinal triangle is bounded laterally by the inferior epigastric artery, medially by the rectus abdominis muscle, and inferiorly by the inguinal ligament. (**Ref. 2,** p. 435)

**191. (C)** The direct or indirect branches of the internal iliac artery are the umbilical, inferior vesical, middle rectal, uterine, vaginal, obturator, internal pudendal, iliolumbar, lateral sacral, superior gluteal, and inferior gluteal. The artery of the ductus deferens is a branch of the umbilical artery. The inferior epigastric artery is a branch of the external iliac artery and supplies the lower abdominal and pelvic wall. (**Ref. 2,** pp. 553–557)

**192. (B)** The superior mesenteric artery supplies the cecum, appendix, ascending colon, right two-thirds of the transverse colon, most of the small intestine, and a portion of the pancreas. The upper portion of the rectum is supplied by the inferior mesenteric artery. (**Ref. 2,** p. 479)

**193. (D)** The epiploic foramen is bounded anteriorly by the right free margin of the lesser omentum, which contains the common bile duct, proper hepatic artery, and portal vein. Posteriorly the epiploic foramen is bounded by the inferior vena cava, inferiorly by the duodenum, and superiorly by the liver. (**Ref. 2,** p. 442)

**194. (C)** The esophageal hiatus passes through the right crus of the diaphragm at the level of the tenth thoracic vertebra. The anterior and posterior vagal trunks enter the abdomen through this hiatus with the esophagus. (**Ref. 2,** pp. 497–499)

**195. (D)** The hepatic portal vein forms posterior to the neck of the pancreas by the confluence of the superior mesenteric and splenic veins. The portal vein ascends in the hepatoduodenal ligament to reach the liver. (**Ref. 2,** pp. 488–489)

**196. (A)** The lymphatics from the testes follow the spermatic cord through the inguinal canal to reach the lumbar nodes along the renal vessels. (**Ref. 2,** p. 545)

**197. (D)** The transversalis fascia lines the entire abdominopelvic cavity and forms an outpouching called the internal spermatic fascia at the deep inguinal ring. (**Ref. 2,** p. 433)

**198. (E)** The levator ani muscle forms the largest part of the pelvic diaphragm. It is divided into three parts, and is the floor of the pelvic cavity separating the pelvis from the ischioanal fossa. It is not part of the inguinal spaces. (**Ref. 2,** pp. 565–566)

**199. (D)** The splenic artery branches from the celiac trunk and courses along the superior surface of the pancreas, where it provides two or three major arteries to the pancreas. The superior mesenteric and gastroduodenal arteries also supply the pancreas. (**Ref. 2,** p. 453)

**200. (A)** The suprarenal glands receive a rich blood supply from the superior, middle, and inferior suprarenal arteries. These arteries are branches of the inferior phrenic and renal arteries and the abdominal aorta, respectively. (**Ref. 2,** p. 497)

**201. (B)** The deep perineal space in the male contains the sphincter urethrae and transverse perineal muscles, membranous urethra, and bulbourethral glands. The prostate gland is superior to the deep perineal space. (**Ref. 2,** p. 519)

**202. (E)** Lymphatic flow from the upper rectum courses through the vessels along the inferior mesenteric artery in the abdomen. The pudendal canal is a split in the obturator internus fascia. The canal crosses the obturator internus muscle and transmits the pudendal nerve and internal pudendal artery, vein, and lymphatics from the lower rectum. (**Ref. 2,** p. 535)

**203. (A)** The perineum receives its motor nerve supply form branches of the pudendal nerve, which innervates both the urogenital and anal triangles. The named branches are the inferior rectal and perineal nerves and the dorsal nerve of the penis (clitoris). (**Ref. 2**, p. 524)

**204. (C)** Posterior to the second part of the duodenum is the hilum of the right kidney. The other structures are not directly related to the second part of the duodenum. (**Ref. 2**, pp. 458–459)

**205. (D)** From the celiac ganglion, postganglionic sympathetic fibers follow the three arterial branches of the celiac trunk: the splenic, left gastric, and common hepatic arteries. These sympathetics innervate the viscera supplied by these three arteries. (**Ref. 2**, p. 505)

**206. (B)** The omental bursa is the lesser peritoneal sac, which is bounded anteriorly by the lesser omentum and the posterior surface of the stomach. It connects via the epiploic foramen with the greater peritoneal sac. (**Ref. 2**, p. 441)

**207. (C)** The deep inguinal ring is the mouth of the outpouching of the transversalis fascia. It is lateral to the inferior epigastric artery and transmits the spermatic cord (round ligament), and is the site of an indirect hernia. (**Ref. 2**, p. 433)

**208. (A)** The pelvic splanchnic nerves are parasympathetic autonomic fibers that derive from the second, third, and fourth sacral spinal cord segments. The fibers supply the pelvic and distal abdominal viscera. (**Ref. 2**, p. 505)

**209. (D)** The round ligament attaches to the lateral surface of the uterus and courses lateral to the deep inguinal ring. The broad ligament sweeps from the anterior and posterior surfaces of the uterus onto the bladder and uterus, forming the vesicouterine and rectouterine pouches, respectively. The broad ligament helps maintain the anteflexed and anteverted position of the uterus. (**Ref. 2**, pp. 533–534)

**210. (D)** The crura of the clitoris or penis attach to the ischiopubic rami on each side, and then enter the body of the clitoris or penis as the corpora cavernosa. **(Ref. 2, pp. 520–522)**

**211. (D)** The vagus nerve provides the parasympathetic innervation of the gut distally to the left third of the transverse colon at the left colic (splenic) flexure. Distal to this point, the pelvic splanchnic nerves provide parasympathetic innervation to the distal gastrointestinal tract and pelvic viscera. **(Ref. 2, p. 504)**

**212. (F)** The splenic artery branches from the celiac trunk and courses to the left along the superior surface of the pancreas, posterior to the body of the stomach. The artery then enters the hilum of the spleen. **(Ref. 2, p. 453)**

**213. (D)** The celiac trunk is one of the three unpaired branches of the abdominal aorta. This trunk branches at the upper border of the first lumbar vertebra and divides into the common hepatic, left gastric, and splenic arteries. **(Ref. 2, pp. 451–452)**

**214. (B)** The proper hepatic artery branches from the common hepatic artery and ascends the hepatoduodenal ligament to reach the porta of the liver. There it divides into the right and left hepatic arteries. The right hepatic branch supplies the gallbladder. **(Ref. 2, p. 453)**

**215. (G)** The left gastroepiploic artery branches from the splenic artery and courses in the greater omentum (gastrocolic ligament) to supply the stomach along its greater curvature. It communicates with the right gastroepiploic artery. **(Ref. 2, p. 453)**

**216. (E)** The left gastric artery branches form the celiac trunk and courses along the lesser curvature of the stomach in the lesser omentum. It supplies branches to the esophagus and stomach. **(Ref. 2, pp. 451–452)**

**217. (C)** The common hepatic artery branches from the celiac trunk and courses to the right along the superior surface of the pancreas. The artery divides into the proper hepatic and gastroduodenal arteries. The proper hepatic artery supplies the liver and the gastroduoderal artery supplies the stomach, duodenum, and pancreas. (**Ref. 2,** p. 452)

**218. (B)** Sepsis, dilatation of retinal veins, and papilloedema as well as ophthalmoplegia all suggest right cavernous sinus thrombosis. Venous drainage by the ophthalmic veins to the cavernous sinus is blocked, the edema causing exophthalmos and pain on the right side of the face. The total ophthalmoplegia involves the oculomotor (III), trochlear (IV), and abducens (VI) nerves, while the pain from the eye and upper lip involves the ophthalmic and maxillary divisions of the trigeminal nerve. (**Ref. 2,** p. 325)

**219. (D)** The only nerve coursing in the lumen of the cavernous sinus the abducens nerve, along with the internal carotid artery. The oculomotor and trochlear and the ophthalmic and maxillary trigeminal divisions course in the lateral wall of the caverous sinus. The sinus receives blood from the ophthalmic veins and drains into the internal jugular bulb directly or indirectly via the petrosal sinuses. (**Ref. 2,** p. 325)

**220. (C)** The straight sinus drains to the confluens of sinuses and has no connection with the cavernous sinus. Venous flow from the face via the angular and ophthalmic veins, and from the pterygoid plexus, comprises the major inflow to the sinus. (**Ref. 2,** p. 324)

**221. (B)** The abducens nerve pursues a lengthy course in the trabeculated lumen of the cavernous sinus, as opposed to the other related nerves, which are in the protection of the lateral wall of the sinus. Thus, the abducens nerve would be the first nerve impaired by pressure in the cavernous sinus. (**Ref. 2,** p. 296)

**222. (D)** The inferior petrosal sinus lies in the floor of the posterior cranial fossa, whereas the tentorium roofs the posterior cranial fossa and contains each of the other sinuses. The inferior petrosal sinus drains the cavernous sinus posteriorly to the internal jugular bulb. (**Ref. 2,** p. 326)

**223. (C)** The superior rectus muscle is being evaluated when the physician asks a patient to abduct the right eye and look superiorly. This muscle is innervated by the oculomotor nerve, and this is the damaged nerve in this case. (**Ref. 2,** p. 293)

**224. (C)** The phrenic nerve is the motor nerve to the diaphragm that is necessary for respiration, and thus has to be saved. The ansa cervicalis and accessory nerve do not innervate muscles with critical functions. The submandibular gland and internal jugular vein can be removed on one side with little consequence. (**Ref. 2,** pp. 218–220)

**225. (E)** The lymphatic vessels of the upper lip and lateral parts of the lower lip drain into the submandibular nodes, while those from the medial part of the lower lip and chin drain into the submental nodes. Each of these sets of nodes drains into the deep cervical nodes, which empty into the thoracic duct on the right. (**Ref. 2,** p. 270)

**226. (D)** The carotid sheath surrounds the common and internal carotid arteries and the vagus nerve, but the external carotid artery is not in the sheath. The external carotid artery leaves the sheath at the upper border of the thyroid cartilage before dividing into its many branches. The ansa cervicalis is embedded in the sheath. (**Ref. 2,** p. 201)

**227. (B)** Branching from the external carotid artery, the lingual artery goes deep to the hyoglossus muscle, which is in the floor of the submandibular triangle. Each of the other structures is located superficial to the hyoglossus muscle and deep to the mylohyoid muscle. (**Ref. 2,** pp. 213–216)

**228. (A)** The prevertebral fascia is posterior to the pretracheal fascia and surrounds the prevertebral muscles. The buccopharyngeal and pretracheal fasciae bound the visceral compartment containing the trachea, larynx, pharynx, and thyroid gland. (**Ref. 2,** p. 226)

**229. (B)** Erb-Duchenne paralysis (Erb's palsy) is caused by the tearing of C-5 and C-6 roots of the brachial plexus. It usually results from a violent separation of the head and neck that damages the superior trunk of the brachial plexus. The damaged nerve fibers (C-5 and C-6) provide motor innervation to muscles of the upper limb and sensory fibers from the lateral side of the limb. (**Ref. 2,** pp. 121–123, 185)

**230. (C)** Absence of abduction at the shoulder joint, flexion at the elbow, and weakness in supination indicate that the suprascapular, axillary, and musculocutaneous nerves are damaged. Fibers of the suprascapular nerve, branching from the superior trunk (C-5 and C-6) of the brachial plexus, are damaged. Fibers of the axillary nerve, branching from the posterior cord of the plexus and containing C-5 and C-6 fibers, are damaged, and fibers of the musculocutaneous nerve, the continuation of the lateral cord containing C-5 and C-6 fibers, are also damaged. **(Ref. 2,** pp. 121–123)

**231. (D)** The musculocutaneous nerve innervates all muscles in the anterior compartment of the arm (elbow flexion and supination). It is formed by anterior fibers of the superior and middle trunks of the brachial plexus and is sensory from the lateral side of the forearm. **(Ref. 2,** p. 130)

**232. (B)** Formation of the trunks of the brachial plexus is the first step in the mingling of nerve fibers from several cord segments and their subsequent redistribution as named terminal branches of the plexus. Motor and sensory fibers of C-5 and C-6 form the superior trunk. **(Ref. 2,** pp. 119–120)

**233. (D)** Although the lateral cord is composed of axons from spinal cord levels C-5, C-6, and C-7, only fibers in C-5 and C-6 form the musculocutaneous nerve. This nerve pierces the coracobrachialis muscle to course in the anterior compartment of the arm. **(Ref. 2,** p. 130)

**234. (A)** Crossing the elbow joint to its insertion on the tuberosity of the radius, the biceps brachii muscle is a strong flexor at the elbow and supinator of the forearm. The muscle arises from two heads of origin on the scapula, and also functions in flexion at the shoulder joint. **(Ref. 2,** p. 125)

**235. (E)** Through the insertion of the deltoid muscle on the deltoid tuberosity of the humerus, and the insertion of the tendon of the supraspinatus muscle on the greater tubercle, these two strong abductors span the shoulder joint. The supraspinatus initiates abduction while the deltoid, as the most powerful abductor, completes this movement, assisted by the supraspinatus. **(Ref. 2,** pp. 94–97)

**236. (A)** The subscapularis muscle is the most powerful medial rotator, spanning the shoulder joint from its extensive origin on the costal scapular surface to insert on the lesser tubercle of the humerus. Being a postaxial muscle, it is innervated by branches of the posterior cord: the upper and lower subscapular nerves. **(Ref. 2, p. 124)**

**237. (B)** The rotator cuff tendons insert on the greater and lesser tubercles of the humerus whereas the deltoid muscle inserts on the deltoid tuberosity. The rotator cuff muscles are very important in stabilizing the humerus and scapula at the shoulder joint. **(Ref. 2, p. 172)**

**238. (C)** Swelling and pain over the index finger indicates infection in the digital fibrous and synovial sheaths enclosing the flexor digitorum superficialis and profundus tendons. The fibrous sheath is a strong covering of the long flexor tendons and synovial sheath. In the index finger, the digital synovial sheath is not directly continuous with the radial bursa of the palm. **(Ref. 2, p. 163)**

**239. (E)** The dense palmar aponeurosis does not allow for swelling, while the loose tissue of the dorsum of the hand does. Also, as mentioned in the answer to Question 238, there is no continuity of the synovial spaces of the index finger and palm. **(Ref. 2, p. 158)**

**240. (B)** The fibrous sheath of the index finger is continuous with the anterior boundary of the thenar space, which is located on the radial side of the central compartment, deep to the palmar aponerurosis. Therefore, any spread of infection from the index finger would first be to the thenar space. **(Ref. 2, p. 158)**

**241. (D)** The flexor pollicis longus tendon is the sole occupant of the radial bursa. The radial bursa is the synovial sheath of this muscle and extends from the flexor retinaculum distally to just proximal to the insertion of the flexor pollicis longus muscle. **(Ref. 2, p. 143)**

**242. (A)** The mediastinal nodes are located along the internal thoracic artery and primarily receive lymphatic drainage from the medial aspect of the mammary gland. The cubital nodes at the elbow receive lymph from the medial hand and some from the lateral hand. The lateral, central, and pectoral axillary nodes receive most of the lymph from the upper limb, with some drainage to the deltopectoral nodes. (**Ref. 2,** p. 369)

243. (**C**) Trauma at the head of the fibula damaged the deep fibular nerve where it divides from the common fibular nerve. The deep fibular nerve enters the anterior compartment of the leg, where it innervates the dorsiflexors of the foot. The nerve then courses deep to the extensor retinaculum onto the dorsum of the foot. There it provides motor innervation to the short extensor muscles of the medial toes, and sensory innervation from the skin between the first and second toes. The patient's normal plantar flexion, toe flexion, and eversion indicated that the common fibular, superficial fibular, and tibial nerves were not damaged. (**Ref. 2,** pp. 621–625)

244. (**A**) The fibularis longus muscle is located in the lateral compartment of the leg and is innervated by the superficial fibular nerve. This muscle and nerve were not involved in the accident. All the other muscles are located in the anterior compartment of the leg or dorsum of the foot, and were affected because these muscles are innervated by the deep fibular nerve. (**Ref. 2,** p. 611)

245. (**E**) The deep puncture wound at the middle of the calf damaged the posterior tibial artery. This vessel descends through the middle of the posterior compartment of the leg deep to the gastrocnemius and soleus muscles. The posterior tibial artery then courses posterior to the medial malleolus to enter the foot. The weak pulse observed at the medial malleolus was caused by decreased blood flow in the posterior tibial artery at the ankle. (**Ref. 2,** p. 619)

246. (**B**) The superficial fibular nerve provides motor innervation to the muscles of the lateral compartment of the leg, and then courses onto the dorsum of the foot, where it is sensory for most of the dorsal surface of the foot except for the skin between the great toe and second toe. This latter area of skin receives its sensory innervation from the deep fibular nerve. (**Ref. 2,** p. 621)

**247. (D)** The dorsalis pedis artery is the continuation of the anterior tibial artery distal to the extensor retinaculum. The dorsal midline of the foot is a routine location at which to evaluate the quality of blood flow by compressing the dorsalis pedis artery against the tarsal bones. (**Ref. 2,** p. 623)

**248. (C)** The tissues of the hip joint and the head and neck of the femur are supplied with blood mainly by branches of the medial and lateral circumflex femoral arteries, lower branches of the inferior gluteal artery, and the artery to the ligamentum capitis femoris, which is a branch of the obturator artery. This last branch is an important source of blood to the head of the femur, and damage to it often results in necrosis of the superior end of the femur. (**Ref. 2,** pp. 601–602)

**249. (A)** One of the major cutaneous nerves that supply the skin of the calf of the leg is the sural branch of the tibial nerve. Damage to the tibial nerve in the gluteal region and surrounding tissues would affect sensory innervation of the posterior leg. The saphenous nerve supplies the medial side of the leg, and the other nerves are cutaneous from the skin of the thigh. (**Ref. 2,** pp. 580–583)

**250. (E)** Medial (internal) rotation of the thigh at the hip joint is not as strong a movement as lateral (external) rotation. The anterior fibers of the gluteus medius and minimus muscles are primarily involved with medial rotation. These two muscles are complemented by the muscles of the medial (adductor) compartment of the thigh. The sartorius muscle is a member of the anterior compartment of the thigh and functions as a lateral rotator of the hip. (**Ref. 2,** pp. 634–635)

**251. (E)** The externally rotated lower limb resulted from loss of tone of the medial rotators of the thigh, as described in the answer to Question 250. The gluteus medius and minimus muscles are innervated by the superior gluteal nerve, and the muscles of the medial compartment of the thigh are innervated by the obturator nerve. (**Ref. 2,** pp. 589–605)

**252. (A)** The primary flexor muscles of the knee are the three hamstring muscles (semitendinosus, semimembranosus, and the long head of the biceps femoris), located in the posterior compartment of the thigh. Plantar flexion of the foot at the ankle joint is the function of muscles in both the superficial and deep posterior compartments of the leg. All of these posterior thigh and leg muscles are innervated by the tibial nerve, which sustained a high injury at the hip and resulted in these muscular deficits. (**Ref. 2,** pp. 595–596)

**253.** **(C)**   Upon passing through the diaphragm, the inferior vena cava ends immediately in the right atrium, having no intrathoracic course. The superior vena cava, esophagus, phrenic nerve, and recurrent laryngeal nerve would all be vulnerable to thoracic damage. (**Ref. 2,** pp. 408–412)

**254.** **(B)**   The left inferior tracheobronchial lymph nodes are unique. Their efferents do not ascend along the left side of the trachea to the left bronchomediastinal lymph trunk, but rather cross over to the right and ascend in lymph channels on the right side of the trachea. Thus, contralateral metastasis of cancer of the left lower lobe of the lung is common. (**Ref. 2,** p. 401)

**255.** **(E)**   If metastasis to the deep cervical nodes has already occurred, thoracic surgery is regarded as inappropriate. These numerous nodes are arranged along the carotid sheath and are far removed from the efferents of the lung. Thus, if they are positive, there has already been metastasis to other organs (brain). (**Ref. 2,** pp. 208–211)

**256.** **(C)**   The thoracic duct is present only on the left side of the neck. It is the main lymphatic channel and drains into the junction of the left internal jugular vein and left subclavian vein. (**Ref. 2,** p. 211)

**257.** **(A)**   Cardiac sensory input courses with the sympathetic fibers and is known to synapse in the dorsal gray of spinal cord segments T-1 to T-4 or T-5. The intercostobrachial nerve is the somatic sensory branch of T-2 and is responsible for the referred pain of angina to the left limb. (**Ref. 2,** pp. 397–398)

**258.** **(E)**   Cardiac afferents pass through upper thoracic chain ganglia and, via white rami communicantes, reach spinal nerves T-1 to

T-4 or T-5 to enter the spinal cord via the dorsal roots of these nerves. (**Ref. 2,** p. 398)

**259. (B)** Constriction of the coronary arteries is known to be a function of parasympathetic vagal fibers. The preganglionic parasympathetic fibers have their cell bodies in the brain, and the postganglionic cell bodies are located in terminal ganglia on the surface of the heart. (**Ref. 2,** p. 398)

**260. (D)** The right vagus and right sympathetic nerves are known primarily to innervate the sinuatrial node. The atrioventricular node receives branches primarily from left vagal and sympathetic fibers. (**Ref. 2,** pp. 396–397)

**261. (A)** The circumflex branch of the left coronary artery runs in the coronary sulcus and mainly supplies the left atrium and the posterior and lateral parts of the left ventricle. It courses with the great cardiac vein and is deep to the coronary sinus. (**Ref. 2,** p. 387)

**262. (E)** Sympathetic afferents from the stomach (and other abdominal viscera) course through the celiac ganglion (without synapse) and join the efferent preganglionic sympathetic fibers of the greater splanchnic nerve. These fibers pass through the chain ganglia with no synapse and through the white rami communicantes. The fibers join the spinal nerves and dorsal roots where their cell bodies are located in the spinal ganglia. The central processes of the fibers enter the spinal cord. The lesser and least splanchnic nerves are primarily involved with the kidneys and gonads. (**Ref. 2,** pp. 502–507)

**263. (D)** The falciform ligament connects the umbilicus with the fissure for the ligamentum teres of the liver, and is not a boundary of the omental bursa. The transverse mesocolon is inferior and the gastrolienal ligament posterior to the omental bursa, and the hepatogastric and hepatoduodenal ligaments are anterior boundaries of the bursa. (**Ref. 2,** p. 467)

**264. (B)** The lienorenal ligament represents a portion of the dorsal mesogastrium that extends between the spleen and left kidney and is not part of the greater omentum. The prenicocolic ligament is the left extension of the gastrocolic ligament that supports the spleen. (**Ref. 2,** pp. 437–442)

**265. (C)** The splenic artery arises from the celiac trunk and courses to the left along the superior border of the pancreas. At the tail of the pancreas, it enters the lienorenal ligament to reach the hilum of the spleen. (**Ref. 2,** p. 453)

**266. (A)** The pancreas, as part of the stomach bed, is separated from the posterior stomach wall only by peritoneum. Also, the left kidney and left suprarenal gland make up the posterior wall of the omental bursa. (**Ref. 2,** p. 441)

**267. (D)** Sensory nerve endings in the peritoneum covering the gallbladder are stimulated by inflammation. Pain is transmitted into spinal cord segments T-7 to T-9, impinging on neurons receiving sensory input from dermatomes T-7 to T-9 which are in the scapular area. This is an example of referred pain. (**Ref. 2,** p. 476)

**268. (B)** The third part of the duodenum, being retroperitoneal and posteroinferior to the level of the gallbladder, would not be easily exposed to gallbladder infection. The liver, transverse colon, first part of the duodenum, and cystic duct are directly related to the gallbladder and would be succeptible to infection. (**Ref. 2,** pp. 458, 470)

**269. (A)** Typically, the cystic artery is a branch of the right hepatic artery, which derives from the proper hepatic artery. The proper hepatic and gastroduodenal arteries are the two terminal branches of the common hepatic artery. (**Ref. 2,** p. 473)

**270. (E)** In the right, free margin of the lesser omentum (hepatoduodenal ligament portion), the common bile duct lies anterior to the portal vein. The proper hepatic artery is to the left of the common bile duct. The common bile duct courses posterior to the duodenum and deep to the head of the pancreas to join the pancreatic duct. (**Ref. 2,** pp. 467–468)

**271. (E)** Injection studies of the internal drainage of the intrahepatic ducts show that the traditional left lobe includes the quadrate lobe and most of the caudate lobe. Only the caudate process of the caudate lobe belongs to the right lobe and drains into the right hepatic bile duct. (**Ref. 2,** pp. 468–470)

**272. (B)** The classical route for an indirect inguinal hernia is through the deep inguinal ring, which is located just lateral to the inferior epigastric artery. The herniated gut descends through the inguinal canal and becomes covered with all the layers of the spermatic cord. The hernia often extends through the superficial inguinal ring to enter the scrotum. The inguinal triangle is medial to the inferior epigastric artery, and is the site of a direct inguinal hernia. (**Ref. 2,** p. 433)

**273. (C)** The ilioinguinal nerve derives from the lumbar plexus and courses through the posterior, lateral, and anterior abdominal walls. Anteriorly, it pierces through the internal abdominal oblique muscle to enter the inguinal canal. The ilioinguinal nerve then courses on the surface of the spermatic cord through the superficial inguinal ring, where it provides nerves to the anterior wall of the scrotum. (**Ref. 2,** p. 515)

**274. (A)** The internal abdominal oblique and transversus abdominis muscles originate in part from the lateral two-thirds and lateral one-third of the inguinal ligament, respectively. The fibers of these two muscles then arch superiorly and medially over the spermatic cord to form the roof of the inguinal canal. (**Ref. 2,** pp. 423–425)

**275. (E)** From the roof of the inguinal canal, the combined fibers of the internal abdominal oblique and transversus abdominis muscles drop inferiorly and posterior to the medial crus of the superficial inguinal ring to insert on the pubic crest. The fused aponeurosis of these two muscles at their insertion is called the falx inguinalis (conjoint tendon). The falx inguinalis borders and gives considerable strength to the medial aspect of the posterior wall of the inguinal canal, thus limiting any gut herniation at this location. (**Ref. 2,** p. 425)

**276. (A)** The pelvic splanchnic nerves comprise the parasympathetic innervation to the gut distal to the splenic flexure of the large colon, which is not involved in an inguinal hernia. Visceral pain from the ileum is carried by nerve fibers that course in the greater, lesser, and least splanchnic nerves, which usually enter the spinal cord in its lowest seven or eight segments. (**Ref. 2,** p. 562)

277. **(C)** The lymphatic channels from the cervix drain laterally across the floor of the pelvis adjacent to the vascular systems in this location. These lymphatic vessels drain mainly into the internal iliac nodes and partly into some of the external iliac nodes. These two lymphatic channels then form the common iliac nodes, which join those from the opposite side of the body at the bifurcation of the aorta to form the lumbar chain of nodes. The lumbar nodes ascend along the abdominal aorta, where they unite and form the lumbar trunk. (**Ref. 2,** p. 551)

278. **(D)** The uterine artery is one of the numerous visceral branches of the internal iliac (hypogastric) artery. The uterine artery courses medially across the floor of the pelvis in the cardinal ligaments to reach the lateral side of the isthmus of the uterus. Approximately 2 centimeters from the uterus, the ureter crosses inferiorly to the artery on its way to the bladder. This close proximity between the uterus and ureter requires careful dissection during ligation of the uterine artery in order to avoid damage to the ureter. (**Ref. 2,** p. 557)

279. **(A)** The broad ligament is divided into anterior and posterior layers as it sweeps over the uterus and attached structures. The round ligament attaches to the lateral surface of the fundus of the uterus just below the attachment of the uterine tubes, and courses anterolaterally in the anterior layer of the broad ligament to enter the deep ring of the inguinal canal. The round ligament can be seen as an elevated fold on the anterior surface of the broad ligament. (**Ref. 2,** pp. 533–534)

280. **(C)** During a radical hysterectomy, great care is given to removing as many as possible of the lymph nodes at the uterus and on the floor and side walls of the pelvis. On the lateral wall of the pelvis and surface of the obturator muscle, the oburator nerve and vessels have to be protected during surgery. The oburator nerve and artery derive from the lumbar plexus and internal iliac artery, respectively, and then course on the lateral pelvic wall, exiting the obturator foramen and canal to supply the muscles of the medial compartment of the thigh. (**Ref. 2,** p. 516)

**281. (B)** The ureters descend the posterior abdominal wall lying on the surface of the psoas major muscle. After being crossed anteriorly by the gonadal vessels, the ureters enter the pelvis by passing over the pelvic brim at the bifurcation of the common iliac arteries. At the brim, the suspensory ligament of the ovary (infundibulopelvic ligament) is adjacent to the lateral side of the ureter. The ligament contains in part the ovarian vessels, which have to be separated from the ureter before they can be ligated. **(Ref. 2, pp. 493–541, 542)**

**282. (E)** The internal iliac artery arises from the common iliac artery at the level of the sacroiliac joint. The initial course of the internal iliac artery is short, and at the level of the greater sciatic foramen a number of posterior branches arise from the artery that are primarily parietal in distribution. The largest and most significant of these posterior branches is the superior gluteal artery, which exits the pelvic floor to supply the gluteal muscles of the hip. **(Ref. 2, pp. 553–557)**

# 2

# Neuroanatomy

---

**DIRECTIONS (Questions 1–69):** Each of the questions or incomplete statements below is followed by five suggested answers or completions. Select the **one** that is best in each case.

---

1. Injury to the medial lemniscus causes
   A. paralysis of extremities on the opposite side
   B. tactile deficits on the opposite side
   C. pain deficits on the same side
   D. temperature deficits on the same side
   E. proprioceptive deficits on the same side

2. All of the nuclei listed below give origin to general somatic efferent fibers **EXCEPT** the
   A. oculomotor
   B. trochlear
   C. abducens
   D. facial
   E. hypoglossal

3. The cerebral arterial circle (circle of Willis) is formed by branches of the internal carotid artery and the
   A. external carotid artery
   B. vertebral artery
   C. basilar artery
   D. middle meningeal artery
   E. anterior temporal artery

4. Each of the following is homologous with spinal ganglia **EXCEPT**
   A. semilunar ganglion
   B. geniculate ganglion
   C. vestibular ganglion
   D. inferior ganglion of the vagus nerve
   E. submandibular ganglion

5. Numerous ascending axons of the reticular formation become a part of the
   A. central tegmental fasciculus
   B. lemniscal system
   C. posterior limb of the internal capsule
   D. medial longitudinal fasciculus
   E. fasciculus retroflexus

6. The important areas nourished by the middle cerebral artery include all of the following **EXCEPT** the
   A. motor areas
   B. premotor areas
   C. primary visual area
   D. somesthetic projection areas
   E. auditory projection areas

7. The cerebral aqueduct is located within the
   A. telencephalon
   B. diencephalon
   C. mesencephalon
   D. metencephalon
   E. myelencephalon

8. The layer of connective tissue immediately adjacent to the brain is known as the
   A. dura mater
   B. arachnoid
   C. pia mater
   D. ependyma
   E. choroid plexus

9. One of the pathways of the extrapyramidal system is the
   A. corticospinal tract
   B. fasciculus proprius
   C. fornix
   D. dorsal white columns
   E. rubrospinal tract

10. Broca's area is located in the
    A. superior temporal gyrus
    B. opercular and triangular parts of the inferior frontal gyrus
    C. precentral gyrus
    D. postcentral gyrus
    E. superior frontal gyrus

11. Each of the following give rise to secretomotor axons **EXCEPT** the
    A. inferior salivatory nucleus
    B. pterygopalatine ganglion
    C. geniculate ganglion
    D. submandibular ganglion
    E. superior cervical ganglion

12. A medullary source of imput to lower motor neurons of the visceral efferent system is the
    A. dorsal longitudinal fasciculus
    B. hypothalamus
    C. mammillary peduncle
    D. reticulospinal tract
    E. mammillotegmental tract

**13.** The primary visual cortex is located in the
   **A.** temporal lobe
   **B.** frontal lobe
   **C.** parietal lobe
   **D.** occipital lobe
   **E.** insula

**14.** The tract of the spinal cord that is specifically related to light touch is the
   **A.** spinotectal tract
   **B.** spino-olivary tract
   **C.** lateral spinothalamic tract
   **D.** anterior spinothalamic tract
   **E.** spinovestibular tract

**15.** The insula is part of the
   **A.** cerebral cortex
   **B.** cerebellar cortex
   **C.** basal ganglia
   **D.** brainstem
   **E.** thalamus

**16.** Functionally, the nucleus of Clark is most closely related to the
   **A.** substantia gelatinosa
   **B.** nucleus gracilis
   **C.** nucleus cuneatus
   **D.** accessory cuneatus nucleus
   **E.** inferior vestibular nucleus

**17.** The structure that separates the globus pallidus from the thalamus is the
   **A.** internal capsule
   **B.** anterior commissure
   **C.** corpus callosum
   **D.** lenticular fasciculus
   **E.** thalamic fasciculus

**18.** The highest probability for the location of the nerve cell body of an axon in the lateral corticospinal tract would be the
   **A.** ipsilateral superior temporal gyrus
   **B.** contralateral inferior temporal gyrus

**C.** ipsilateral precentral gyrus
**D.** contralateral precentral gyrus
**E.** contralateral postcentral gyrus

19. The medial lemniscus is in part derived from fibers of the
    **A.** gracilis and cuneate nuclei of the same side
    **B.** gracilis and cuneate nuclei of the opposite side
    **C.** gracilis nucleus of the same side and the cuneate nucleus of the opposite side
    **D.** gracilis nucleus of the opposite side and the cuneate nucleus of the same side
    **E.** ventral posterolateral nucleus of the thalamus

20. An injury of the lateral spinothalamic tract would be expected to result in loss of pain and temperature sensation
    **A.** one segment below the level of the lesion on the ipsilateral side
    **B.** one segment below the level of the lesion on the contralateral side
    **C.** gradually over several segments below the level of the lesion on the contralateral side
    **D.** two segments below the level of the lesion on the ipsilateral side
    **E.** two segments below the level of the lesion on the contralateral side

21. Lesion of the alpha motor neurons in the anterior horn results in
    **A.** fibrillation
    **B.** flaccid paralysis
    **C.** recruitment
    **D.** myotonic discharge
    **E.** paresthesia

22. The ventral lateral nucleus of the thalamus is an important synaptic site for fibers from the
    **A.** cerebellum and basal ganglia
    **B.** medial lemniscus
    **C.** superior colliculus
    **D.** amygdala and hypothalamus
    **E.** thalamus

**23.** The thalamic nucleus that projects to the prefrontal cortex and is involved in prefrontal functions of foresight is the
  **A.** pulvinar
  **B.** anterior nucleus
  **C.** ventral lateral nucleus
  **D.** ventral anterior nucleus
  **E.** dorsomedial nucleus

**24.** Axons of the lenticular fasciculus project mainly to the
  **A.** medial geniculate body
  **B.** striatum
  **C.** thalamus
  **D.** red nucleus
  **E.** substantia nigra

**25.** In amyotrophic lateral sclerosis
  **A.** both anterior horn alpha motor neurons and lateral corticospinal tracts are affected
  **B.** the anterior horn alpha motor neurons alone are affected
  **C.** the lateral corticospinal tracts alone are affected
  **D.** the lateral corticospinal tracts and dorsal root ganglia are affected
  **E.** the dorsomedial nucleus of the thalamus is affected

**26.** The thalamic fasciculus contains
  **A.** efferent axons from the globus pallidus
  **B.** efferent axons from the red nucleus and globus pallidus
  **C.** efferent axons from the globus pallidus, red nucleus, and dentate nucleus
  **D.** efferent axons from the red nucleus and dentate nucleus
  **E.** efferent axons from the dentate nucleus

**27.** The passageway between the third and lateral ventricles of the brain is called the
  **A.** lateral recess of Magendie
  **B.** aqueduct of Sylvius
  **C.** interventricular foramen of Monro
  **D.** foramen of Luschka
  **E.** rhomboid fossa

28. The medial surfaces of the frontal, parietal, and limbic lobes are supplied by the
    A. middle cerebral artery
    B. anterior cerebral artery
    C. anterior communicating artery
    D. posterior cerebral artery
    E. anterior choroidal artery

29. Parasympathic preganglionic cell bodies found in the superior salivatory nucleus of the pons supply the
    A. lacrimal gland
    B. sublingual gland
    C. submandibular gland
    D. parotid gland
    E. nasal mucous glands

30. The gray matter is composed of each of the following **EXCEPT**
    A. nerve cells
    B. unmyelinated axons
    C. myelinated axons
    D. capillaries
    E. fiber tracts

31. A fluent (receptive) aphasia is best correlated with a lesion of the
    A. left frontal lobe
    B. right frontal lobe
    C. left parietal lobe
    D. left occipital lobe
    E. right thalamus

32. All of the following neuronal structures are a part of the cochlear pathway **EXCEPT** the
    A. spiral ganglion
    B. medial longitudinal fasciculus
    C. cochlear nuclei
    D. lateral lemniscus
    E. medial geniculate body

**33.** Ascending tracts and fibers of the spinal cord include the
   **A.** anterior spinothalamic
   **B.** corticospinal
   **C.** spinotectal
   **D.** spino-olivary
   **E.** spinoreticular

**34.** Pathways crossing in the spinal cord mediate each of the following **EXCEPT**
   **A.** pain
   **B.** temperature
   **C.** muscle tone
   **D.** touch
   **E.** sensory impulses from tendons

**35.** The motor nucleus of the facial nerve is located in the
   **A.** spinal cord
   **B.** medulla oblongata
   **C.** pons
   **D.** mesencephalon
   **E.** thalamus

**36.** The anterior spinothalamic tract conveys impulses of
   **A.** cold
   **B.** pain
   **C.** muscle tone
   **D.** heat
   **E.** light touch

**37.** The vestibulospinal tract is composed of fibers derived from the
   **A.** superior vestibular nucleus
   **B.** inferior olivary nucleus
   **C.** inferior vestibular nucleus
   **D.** lateral vestibular nucleus
   **E.** spinal trigeminal tract

**38.** A major source of afferent stimulation to the substantia nigra is the
   **A.** thalamus
   **B.** caudate nucleus
   **C.** cerebellum

**D.** red nucleus
**E.** hypothalamus

39. The cerebellum is associated with each of the following **EXCEPT**
   **A.** programming of rapid, skilled voluntary movements
   **B.** integration of proprioception with reflex activity
   **C.** coordination of somatic motor activity
   **D.** regulation of muscle tone
   **E.** tactile sense appreciation

40. The pontine nuclei are continuous with which nucleus of the medulla oblongata?
   **A.** arcuate nucleus
   **B.** lateral reticular nucleus
   **C.** hypoglossal nucleus
   **D.** vagal nucleus
   **E.** spinal vestibular nucleus

41. Which of the following nuclear masses is associated with the trigeminal nerve?
   **A.** nucleus of the spinal tract
   **B.** principal sensory nucleus
   **C.** motor nucleus
   **D.** mesencephalic nucleus
   **E.** nucleus ambiguus

42. The basal ganglia include each of the following **EXCEPT** the
   **A.** caudate nucleus
   **B.** red nucleus
   **C.** putamen
   **D.** globus pallidus
   **E.** substantia nigra

43. The human cerebellum receives both primary and secondary vestibular fibers via the juxtarestiform body. These axons terminate mainly in the
   **A.** anterior lobe
   **B.** flocculus
   **C.** posterior lobe
   **D.** vernal region of the corpus cerebelli
   **E.** paravermal or intermediate region of the corpus cerebelli

**44.** The axons that comprise the optic nerves and tracts arise from neuronal soma located in the retina called
  A.  rods and cones
  B.  bipolar cells
  C.  pigmented cells
  D.  ganglion cells
  E.  amacrine cells

**45.** In the human it appears probable that olfactory stimuli reach the primary olfactory cortex directly via the
  A.  anterior commissure
  B.  medial olfactory stria
  C.  diagonal band of Broca
  D.  intermediate olfactory stria and olfactory tubercle
  E.  lateral olfactory stria

**46.** The epithalamus includes each of the following **EXCEPT** the
  A.  pineal body
  B.  roof of the third ventricle
  C.  subthalamus
  D.  stria medullaris
  E.  habenular commissure

**47.** The optic chiasma and tuber cinereum are parts of the
  A.  thalamus
  B.  epithalamus
  C.  subthalamus
  D.  hypothalamus
  E.  pons

**48.** Hypothalamic lesions often cause each of the following **EXCEPT**
  A.  dysmetria
  B.  somnolence
  C.  disturbances of temperature regulation
  D.  disturbances of fat metabolism
  E.  disturbances in eating habits

**49.** Commissure fibers joining the cerebral hemispheres are located in the
  A.  inferior colliculus
  B.  corpus callosum

C. stria medullaris
D. striae terminalis
E. medial lemniscus

50. Connecting the orbital gyri of the frontal lobe with the rostral part of the temporal lobe is the
   A. superior occipitofrontal fasciculus
   B. superior longitudinal fasciculus
   C. cingulum
   D. uncinate fasciculus
   E. putamen

51. The function of the hippocampus is
   A. taste
   B. smell
   C. memory
   D. sight
   E. motor control

52. Posteriorly, the floor of the lateral ventricle is formed by the
   A. caudate nucleus
   B. hippocampus
   C. amygdaloid nuclear complex
   D. septum pellucidum
   E. thalamus

53. The medial forebrain bundle connects the limbic system (septal area) with the
   A. epithalamus
   B. hypothalamus
   C. finely myelinated fibers of the hippocampus
   D. orbital cortex
   E. retina

54. The cerebellum receives afferent impulses from each of the following EXCEPT the
   A. spinal cord
   B. medulla oblongata
   C. pons
   D. cerebrum
   E. hypothalamus

55. The superior cerebellar peduncle consists partly of efferent fibers derived from the
    A. dentate nucleus
    B. red nucleus
    C. amygdaloid nucleus
    D. cuneate nucleus
    E. inferior olivary nucleus

56. The Purkinje cells of the cerebellum are described by each of the following **EXCEPT** they
    A. have large cell bodies
    B. are arranged in a continuous sheet
    C. are difficult to stain
    D. have axons that enter white matter
    E. have elaborate dendritic arborizations

57. Each of the following is correct concerning the structure of the thalamus **EXCEPT**
    A. the third ventricle separates the two thalami
    B. the dorsal surface is covered by the stratum zonale
    C. the external medullary lamina is on the lateral surface
    D. the dorsomedial nucleus is contained therein
    E. it is composed of white matter

58. Each of the following are layers of the dentate gyrus or hippocampus **EXCEPT** the
    A. molecular layer
    B. Purkinje layer
    C. granular layer
    D. polymorphic layer
    E. pyramidal layer

59. The principal cell types found in the cerebral neocortex are pyramidal neurons and the
    A. stellate cells
    B. fusiform cells
    C. Purkinje cells
    D. pyramidal cells
    E. cells of Martinotti

**60.** Corticobulbar axons terminate on all of the following motor nuclei **EXCEPT** the
- **A.** nucleus ambiguus
- **B.** Edinger–Westphal nucleus
- **C.** hypoglossal motor nucleus (cranial nerve XII)
- **D.** motor nucleus of cranial nerve V (masticator nucleus)
- **E.** facial motor nucleus (cranial nerve VII)

**61.** A major site of synapse for axons of the giant pyramidal cells (of Betz) is
- **A.** alpha anterior horn cells
- **B.** red nucleus
- **C.** inferior olivary nuclear complex
- **D.** facial motor nucleus (cranial nerve VII)
- **E.** gamma anterior horn cells

**62.** The largest concentration of centers controlling visceral functions is located in the
- **A.** septal area
- **B.** amygdaloid nuclear complex
- **C.** hippocampal formation
- **D.** hypothalamus
- **E.** motor cortex

**63.** Each of the following is an established primary sensory area in the cerebral cortex **EXCEPT** the
- **A.** visual area
- **B.** somatosensory area
- **C.** auditory area
- **D.** thermal area
- **E.** olfactory area

**64.** The inferior cerebellar peduncle contains
- **A.** fibers of the posterior spinocerebellar tract
- **B.** fibers of the corticopontine tract
- **C.** ventral external arcuate fibers
- **D.** fibers of the ventral spinocerebellar tract
- **E.** fibers to the red nucleus

**65.** Each of the following masses of gray matter is within the cerebral hemispheres **EXCEPT** the
   A. caudate nucleus
   B. lenticular nucleus
   C. amygdaloid nucleus
   D. claustrum
   E. globose nucleus

**66.** Patients with diseased basal ganglia exhibit each of the following **EXCEPT**
   A. the parkinsonian syndrome
   B. athetosis
   C. aphasia
   D. chorea
   E. ballismus

**67.** The hippocampus is
   A. concerned with recent memory
   B. fused with the parahippocampal gyrus
   C. related to olfactory function
   D. located in the roof of the superior horn of the lateral ventricle
   E. part of the occipital lobe

**68.** Uncinate fits are preceded by
   A. transient loss of vision
   B. visual hallucinations
   C. a sense of unreality
   D. disagreeable olfactory sensations
   E. auditory hallucinations

**69.** Each of the following is associated with the temporal lobe **EXCEPT**
   A. auditory impulses
   B. visual impulses
   C. gustatory impulses
   D. olfactory impulses
   E. memory recall

DIRECTIONS (Questions 70–74): Each group of questions below consists of five lettered headings followed by a list of numbered words or statements. For each numbered word or statement, select the **one** lettered heading that is most closely associated with it. Each lettered heading may be selected once, more than once, or not at all.

    **A.** vagus nerve
    **B.** hypoglossal nerve
    **C.** trigeminal nerve
    **D.** facial nerve
    **E.** oculomotor nerve

**70.** Contains proprioceptive fibers from cells of origin in the mesencephalic nucleus.

**71.** Has special visceral efferent fibers from the nucleus ambiguus.

**72.** Has its nucleus of origin in the central gray of the medial eminence in the floor of the fourth ventricle.

**73.** Its dorsal cell column innervates the inferior rectus muscle.

**74.** Contains special visceral efferent and parasympathetic fibers.

DIRECTIONS (Questions 75–81): Identify the structures described in the numbered statements below on the schematic transverse section of the medulla. (Figure 7)

**75.** A lesion of this structure would result in ipsilateral paralysis of the tongue muscles.

**76.** Contains afferent fibers from the vestibular ganglion.

**77.** Conducts the primary ipsilateral afferent fibers from the spinal cord to the cerebellum.

**78.** Bilateral, thick fiber bundles in the medulla that contain descending pathways from the precentral gyrus of the cerebral cortex.

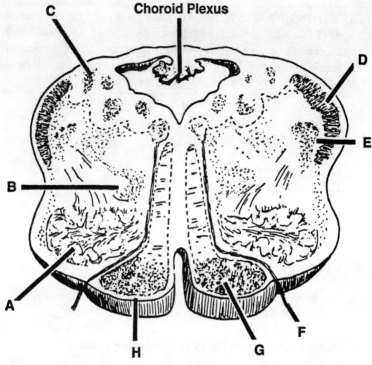

**Figure 7** Transverse section of medulla (From Wilson JE. *Anatomy*, 9th ed. New York: Elsevier, 1991, p. 185.)

**79.** Receives most of its afferent fibers from the ipsilateral red nucleus.

**80.** Gives origin to special visceral efferent fibers that innervate most of the pharyngeal musculature.

**81.** Receives afferent fibers that are responsible for the transmission of most of the tactile, pain, and temperature modalities from the head.

**DIRECTIONS (Questions 82–86):** Identify the structures on the schematic frontal section through the pons (Figure 8).

**82.** Is part of the reticular formation and receives projections from the cerebellar nuclei and from the precentral and premotor cerebral cortices.

**83.** Interconnects homologous areas between the two cerebral hemispheres.

**84.** Lesions that compress the walls of the third ventricle could affect the blood supply to this structure.

**85.** A lesion in this structure can affect muscular movements through its influence on the motor areas of the cerebral cortex.

**86.** A pigmented (melanin) band of gray matter in the tegmentum concerned with muscle tone.

**Figure 8** Frontal section through the pons. (Modified from Frick H et al.: *Human Anatomy I,* Stuttgart: George Thieme Verlag, 1991.)

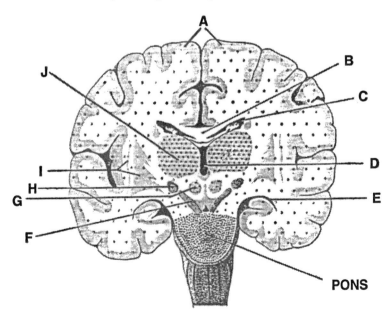

**DIRECTIONS (Questions 87–128):** Each of the case studies below is followed by numbered questions or incomplete statements. Select the **one** best letter answer for each numbered question.

## Case Study I:

A 55-year-old woman was referred because of numbness in the legs. Two years earlier she had begun using a cane because her gait was unsteady. One year ago she stopped driving because of an inability to feel the gas pedal and brake. Recently, the numbness spread to involve her hands. For the last year she had complained of sudden sharp pains of 1 to 2 seconds duration, variable in location, but usually localized to one or the other leg. She had seen several physicians, had a work-up for diabetes mellitus that was negative, and received vitamin $B_{12}$ injections with no benefit.

On examination she showed normal mental status. Her pupils were of unequal size, with the right 3.5 mm and the left 1.5 mm. The left pupil was irregular. Corrected visual acuity was 20/30 bilaterally. The right pupil reacted slowly to light and accommodation; the left pupil accommodated but did not react to light. The cranial nerves were otherwise normal. The patient's strength was normal. Romberg's sign was present (positive). The patient was areflexic in all limbs. Position sense and vibratory perception were reduced in the arms and absent in the legs. Light touch, pain, and temperature perception were normal. The patient's gait was grossly ataxic, broad-based, and slapping.

**87.** The most likely diagnosis is
   A. Brown–Séquard syndrome
   B. tabes dorsalis
   C. multiple sclerosis
   D. meningioma
   E. syringomyelia

**88.** The Argyll–Robertson pupils suggest a lesion in the
   A. optic nerve
   B. Edinger–Westphal nucleus
   C. oculomotor nerve
   D. ciliary ganglion
   E. pretectal region

**89.** A positive Romberg's sign indicates
   **A.** spinocerebellar degeneration
   **B.** upper motor neuron damage
   **C.** posterior column disease
   **D.** optic nerve degeneration
   **E.** lower motor neuron damage

**90.** The ataxia results from
   **A.** loss of ventral horn motor neurons
   **B.** loss of position sense and vibratory perception
   **C.** damage to the ventral roots
   **D.** cerebellar damage
   **E.** damage to the corticospinal tracts

**91.** The areflexia is the result of
   **A.** denegeration of lower motor neurons
   **B.** cerebellar disease
   **C.** damage to the corticospinal tracts
   **D.** degeneration in the posterior columns
   **E.** degeneration in the lateral funiculus

# Case Study II:

A 52-year-old man suddenly felt giddy and faint. He got up from his chair, turned pale, then fell on his right side. He seemed unconscious for a few minutes but soon recognized people in the room and began to speak with his usual distinctness. He was seen a few hours later by a physician who found a paralysis on the right side from face to toes, ptosis of the left upper eyelid, and a left external strabismus.

Neurologic examination 2 days later showed ptosis of the left upper eyelid. The left eye was turned laterally and slightly downward, and the patient was unable to move the left eye medially. The left pupil was dilated and not responsive to light or accommodation. There was paralysis of the muscles of the lower face on the right side. On protrusion, the tip of the tongue turned slightly to the right. A spastic right hemiplegia was present. Both limbs were hypertonic and hyperreflexic, and Babinski's sign was present (positive) on the right. Superficial reflexes were absent.

**92.** A likely diagnosis is
  A. Weber's syndrome
  B. middle alternating hemiplegia
  C. Benedikt's syndrome
  D. Horner's syndrome
  E. Millard–Gubler syndrome

**93.** The emerging oculomotor nerve lies on the crus cerebri in close proximity to the
  A. posterior inferior cerebellar artery
  B. posterior communicating artery
  C. anterior inferior cerebellar artery
  D. posterior cerebral artery
  E. middle cerebral artery

**94.** Paralysis of the right lower facial muscles and turning of the tongue to the right on protrusion indicate involvement of
  A. axons of the right corticospinal tract
  B. axons of the left and right corticobulbar tracts
  C. axons of the left corticobulbar tract
  D. axons of the left corticospinal tract
  E. axons of the right corticobulbar tract

**95.** The Babinski sign is
  A. inability to touch the nose with the index finger (eyes closed)
  B. flexion of the great toe and the four lateral toes
  C. loss of pain and temperature perception
  D. diagnostic of posterior column disease
  E. extension of the great toe and fanning of the four lateral toes

**96.** Upper motor neuron damage is characterized by
  A. hypotonia and flaccid paralysis
  B. spastic paralysis, absence of superficial reflexes, and a Babinski sign
  C. Romberg's sign
  D. degeneration in the posterior columns
  E. damage to the spinothalamic tracts

**97.** Elevation of the upper eyelid and constriction of the pupil are a function of

   **A.** the abducens nerve

   **B.** the facial nerve

   **C.** the oculomotor nerve

   **D.** sympathetic innervation

   **E.** the trigeminal nerve

## Case Study III:

A 63-year-old man with known hypertension awoke to find that his gait was unsteady and that he had numbness on the right side of his face. No paralysis was present. He was alert and his speech was fluent, although his voice was hoarse. The patient had difficulty in swallowing, slight ptosis of the right eyelid, and constriction of the right pupil. There was diminished pain and temperature perception on the right side of the face and on the left side of the body below the head. Ataxia and hypotonia were present in the right limbs and there was a tendency to fall to the right.

    Neurologic examination showed paralysis of the right soft palate (the uvula was deviated to the left and there was poor elevation of the right soft palate). There was paralysis of the right vocal cord, and the gag reflex was absent. Horner's syndrome was present on the right, consisting of slight ptosis of the upper eyelid, constriction of the pupil, anhidrosis, and enophthalmos. Testing of the motor system revealed ataxia in the use of the right limbs, as well as hypotonia. Sensory examination revealed decreased pain and temperature perception on the right side of the face and on the left side of the body below the head.

**98.** The most likely location of the lesion in this case is the

   **A.** ventrolateral medulla

   **B.** ventromedial pons

   **C.** lateral pons

   **D.** dorsolateral medulla

   **E.** ventromedial medulla

**99.** The most likely diagnosis is
    **A.** Millard–Gubler syndrome
    **B.** Wallenberg's syndrome
    **C.** Benedikt's syndrome
    **D.** Guillain–Barré syndrome
    **E.** Weber's syndrome

**100.** The ataxia and hypotonia suggest damage to the
    **A.** nucleus ambiguus
    **B.** spinal trigeminal tract
    **C.** lateral spinothalamic tract
    **D.** spinal trigeminal nucleus
    **E.** inferior cerebellar peduncle

**101.** The slight ptosis of the upper eyelid characteristic of Horner's syndrome is caused by dysfunction of the
    **A.** levator palpebrae superioris muscle
    **B.** orbicularis oculi muscle
    **C.** Muller's tarsal muscle
    **D.** frontalis muscle
    **E.** superior oblique muscle

**102.** Axons from this region, descending in the dorsolateral brain stem tegmentum to reach preganglionic sympathetic neurons of the intermediolateral cell column, produce Horner's syndrome when interrupted
    **A.** hypothalamus
    **B.** epithalamus
    **C.** basal ganglia
    **D.** thalamus
    **E.** cerebral cortex

**103.** The loss of pain and temperature sensation over the right side of the face and left side of the body below the head occurs because the
    **A.** lateral spinothalamic tract crosses at brain stem levels
    **B.** trigeminothalamic tract crosses at brain stem levels
    **C.** lateral spinothalamic tract crosses at spinal levels
    **D.** trigeminothalamic tracts are not crossed
    **E.** trigeminothalamic tracts cross at spinal levels

104. Muller's tarsal muscle is innervated by the
   A. oculomotor nerve
   B. sympathetic system
   C. facial nerve
   D. trigeminal nerve
   E. parasympathetic system

105. The etiology in this case is probably occlusion of the
   A. left vertebral artery
   B. right posterior superior cerebellar artery
   C. right superior cerebellar artery
   D. right vertebral artery or right posterior inferior cerebellar artery
   E. posterior inferior cerebellar artery

# Case Study IV:

A 45-year-old male vagrant was admitted showing confusion, confabulation, amnesia, and disorientation. He said he was alcoholic and had been drinking heavily for years. Blood and cerebrospinal fluid showed alcohol to be present.

Neurologic examination showed ataxia in both lower extremeties, foot drop, and general paresis. Areflexia was present in the lower limbs at the ankle and knee, and lower limb muscles and nerves were painful when squeezed.

106. The mental symptoms are indicative of
   A. Kluver–Bucy syndrome
   B. Korsakoff's syndrome
   C. myasthenia gravis
   D. alexia
   E. Wernicke's syndrome

107. The peripheral nerve involvement is caused by
   A. tabes dorsalis
   B. amyotrophic lateral sclerosis
   C. Alzheimer's disease
   D. muscular dystrophy
   E. polyneuritis

**108.** Each of the following is part of the limbic system **EXCEPT** the
- **A.** inferior cerebellar peduncle
- **B.** amygdala
- **C.** parahippocampal gyrus
- **D.** mammillary bodies
- **E.** hippocampus

**109.** The etiology in this case is very likely
- **A.** dopamine deficiency
- **B.** bacterial infection
- **C.** genetic
- **D.** thiamine deficiency
- **E.** viral infection

**110.** Each of the following is a part of the limbic lobe **EXCEPT** the
- **A.** uncus
- **B.** subcallosal gyrus
- **C.** mammillary bodies
- **D.** cingulate gyrus
- **E.** parahippocampal gyrus

**111.** A frequent site of lesions in Korsakoff's syndrome is the
- **A.** cerebellum
- **B.** mammillary bodies
- **C.** amydala
- **D.** globus pallidus
- **E.** cerebral cortex

## Case Study V:

A 63-year-old woman shows a fine, pill-rolling tremor in both upper extremities, which is tremor at rest. The face is unexpressive and the eyes staring, blinking infrequently. There is an overall poverty of movement, particularly association movements. The patient's gait is shuffling and motor performance is delayed.

**112.** The most likely diagnosis is
- **A.** Wilson's disease
- **B.** Parkinson's disease
- **C.** Benedikt's syndrome

**D.** Liver-brain disease
**E.** Gerstman's syndrome

**113.** Dysfunction of this structure is implicated in Parkinson's disease
  **A.** substantia gelatinosa
  **B.** red nucleus
  **C.** substantia nigra
  **D.** cerebellum
  **E.** substantia innominata

**114.** In Parkinson's disease, there is insufficient production or release of
  **A.** norepinephrine
  **B.** acetylcholine
  **C.** serotonin
  **D.** adrenalin
  **E.** dopamine

**115.** An important neural connection in Parkinson's disease is the projection of the substantia nigra to the
  **A.** corpus striatum
  **B.** amygdala
  **C.** claustrum
  **D.** hypothalamus
  **E.** septal area

**116.** Treatment for Parkinson's disease involves administration of
  **A.** dopamine
  **B.** L-dihydroxyphenyalanine (L-dopa)
  **C.** acetylcholine
  **D.** norepinephrine
  **E.** serotonin

# Case Study VI:

A 40-year-old man became unconscious while inspecting a poorly ventilated conduit into which some natural gas had escaped. He remained unconscious after being carried out into fresh air. Several days passed before he became alert enough to make an accurate neurologic examination possible.

Neurologic examination showed diplopia and a right internal strabismus. Hypertonia and an increase in deep tendon reflexes (hypertonicity) were present on the left, but superficial reflexes (abdominal, cremaster) were absent. The Babinski sign was present on the left. Only gross voluntary movements of the left upper and lower extremities were possible.

117. The right internal strabismus indicates damage to the
    A. oculomotor nerve
    B. trochlear nerve
    C. facial nerve
    D. trigeminal nerve
    E. abducens nerve

118. Hypertonia, hyperreflexia, and a Babinski sign in the left extremities suggest damage to the
    A. left corticobulbar tract
    B. right corticospinal tract
    C. right corticobulbar tract
    D. posterior columns
    E. left corticospinal tract

119. The most likely diagnosis is
    A. inferior alternating hemiplegia
    B. Benedikt's syndrome
    C. superior alternating hemiplegia
    D. middle alternating hemiplegia
    E. oculomotor nerve palsy

120. The lesion site in this case is in the
    A. lateral medulla
    B. basilar pons
    C. lateral mesencephalon
    D. medial medulla
    E. rostral pons

121. Gross postural movements are possible through the influence of the
    A. extrapyramidal motor system
    B. corticobulbar system
    C. rubrospinal tract

**D.** corticospinal tract

**E.** cerebellum

**122.** The patient's syndrome is probably caused by occlusion of the
   **A.** anterior inferior cerebellar artery
   **B.** posterior cerebral artery
   **C.** paramedian branches of the basilar artery
   **D.** posterior inferior cerebellar artery
   **E.** vertebral artery

## Case Study VII:

A 69-year-old man presents with a left hemiplegia, left hemianesthesia, and left homonymous hemianopsia, and a diminution of hearing most marked on the left side.

Neurologic examination reveals a loss of pain, temperature, and proprioceptive sensation on the entire left side of the body. Asterognosis is present, as are hypertonia and hyperreflexia in the left extremeties. The Babinski sign is present on the left. Superficial reflexes are absent.

**123.** The extensive motor and sensory loss in this case suggest a lesion in the
   **A.** claustrum
   **B.** right posterior limb of the internal capsule
   **C.** left anterior limb of the internal capsule
   **D.** right external capsule
   **E.** genu of the internal capsule

**124.** Geniculocalcarine (optic radiation) fibers occupy this part of the posterior limb of the internal capsule
   **A.** sublenticular part
   **B.** inferior thalamic peduncle
   **C.** anterior thalamic peduncle
   **D.** retrolenticular part
   **E.** caudatothalamic part

**125.** Ventral-tier thalamic nuclei project to the cerebral cortex through the
   A. superior thalamic peduncle
   B. posterior thalamic peduncle
   C. inferior thalamic peduncle
   D. anterior thalamic peduncle
   E. genu

**126.** Geniculotemporal (auditory radiation) fibers occupy this part of the posterior limb of the internal capsule
   A. anterior thalamic peduncle
   B. retrolenticular part
   C. genu
   D. posterior thalamic peduncle
   E. sublenticular part

**127.** The most likely cause of the findings in this case is
   A. occlusion of the medial striate arteries
   B. occlusion of the anterior cerebral artery
   C. occlusion of the posterior choroidal artery
   D. occlusion of the anterior choroidal artery
   E. occlusion of the posterior cerebral artery

**128.** Corticospinal tract axons occupy the
   A. anterior limb
   B. posterior thalamic peduncle
   C. posterior limb
   D. inferior thalamic peduncle
   E. external capsule

---

**DIRECTIONS (Questions 129–135):** Match the items listed below with the statements given below:

---

   A. lateral lemniscus
   B. globus pallidus
   C. optic tract
   D. putamen
   E. Broca's area 44
   F. optic chiasm
   G. pineal body

H. locus ceruleus
I. Broadman's area 17
J. medial lemniscus
K. hypophysis
L. dentate gyrus
M. optic nerve
N. temporal lobe
O. caudate nucleus
P. dendate nucleus

## Statements:

**129.** Lesions here result in impairment of recent memory.

**130.** Lesions here eliminate or reduce rapid eye movement (REM; paradoxical) sleep.

**131.** A lesion here would result in degenerated axon terminals in the red nucleus.

**132.** A lesion here results in homonymous quadrantic defects in the upper visual field.

**133.** If a lesion occurs here, a diminution in hearing occurs.

**134.** A lesion here interferes with the synthesis of melatonin.

**135.** A lesion here results in loss of motor speech.

# Neuroanatomy

## Answers and Comments

1. **(B)** The internal arcuate fibers decussate and form an ascending bundle known as the medial lemniscus. The crossing over of the medial lemniscus provides a portion of the sensory representation of half the body in the contralateral cerebral cortex. Consequently, an injury to the medial lemniscus will result in loss of tactile and kinesthetic sensation on the contralateral side of the body. (**Ref. 1,** pp. 116–119)

2. **(D)** The general somatic efferent fibers of the oculomotor, trochlear, and abducens nerves supply extraocular muscles. Those of the hypoglossal nerve supply somatic skeletal muscle of the tongue. The facial nerve does not have somatic efferent fibers (**Ref. 1,** p. 135)

3. **(C)** The cerebral arterial circle is formed by the posterior cerebral artery, a branch of the basilar artery, and by the posterior and anterior communicating and anterior cerebral arteries, which are branches of the internal carotid artery. (**Ref. 1,** pp. 440–441)

4. **(E)** The submandibular ganglion is a collection of cell bodies of postganglionic visceral efferent neurons of the chorda tympani nerve, a branch of the facial nerve. All of the other ganglia listed are sensory ganglia. (**Ref. 1,** p. 172)

**5. (E)** The primary long ascending pathway of the brainstem reticular formation is the central tegmental fasciculus. This is a large composite bundle that also contains descending fibers. At the level of the diencephalon this fasciculus projects into the subthalamic region and to the intralaminar nuclei of the thalamus. (**Ref. 1**, pp. 212-214)

**6. (C)** The middle cerebral artery supplies the motor and premotor areas, the somesthetic and auditory projection areas, and the higher receptive associations. The posterior cerebral artery supplies the primary visual area. (**Ref. 1**, pp. 443-445)

**7. (C)** The mesencephalon or midbrain contains a narrow cavity called the cerebral aqueduct, which connects the third and fourth ventricles (**Ref. 1**, p. 192)

**8. (C)** The pia mater is the innermost of the three connective-tissue coverings of the brain. It is adherent to and follows closely the contours of the brain. (**Ref. 1**, p. 2)

**9. (E)** Fibers of the rubrospinal tract arise from cells in the red nucleus located in the central part of the mesencephalic tegmentum. These fibers are given off from the red nucleus, cross the median raphe, and descend to spinal levels. (**Ref.1**, pp. 239-240)

**10. (B)** Broca's area occupies the opercular and triangular parts of the inferior frontal gyrus. This area is involved with language use, and damage to Broca's area results in motor, or expressive, aphasia in which the patient will produce only a few words and have difficulty producing them. (**Ref. 1**, p. 26)

**11. (C)** The geniculate ganglion is the sensory ganglion of cranial nerve VII, and is involved with all sensory functions of the facial nerve. All of the other structures listed are involved with the secretomotor innervation of glands. (**Ref. 1**, p. 171)

**12. (D)** The reticulospinal tracts arise partly from the medullary reticular formation and descend in the lateral funiculus. These fibers are a major alternate route by which lower motor neurons are controlled. (**Ref. 1**, pp. 239-240)

**13. (D)** The occipital lobe is divided by the calcarine sulcus into the cuneus and lingual gyrus. The cortex on both sides of the calcarine sulcus represents the primary visual cortex. The visual cortex receives impulses from the temporal half of the ipsilateral retina and the nasal half of the contralateral retina. (**Ref. 1, p. 405**)

**14. (D)** The anterior spinothalamic tract conducts impulses concerned with "light touch" to higher levels of the neuraxis. Light touch is elicited by stroking an area of skin lacking hair. (**Ref. 1, pp. 86–88**)

**15. (A)** The insula is a part of the cerebral cortex that lies deep in the lateral sulcus and can be seen only when the frontal and temporal lobes are separated. Its fiber connections are incompletely known, but it is believed to be associated with visceral functions. (**Ref. 1, p. 29**)

**16. (D)** The accessory cuneate nucleus is a group of large cells in the dorsolateral part of the medulla, with cytologic features quite similar to those of the nucleus of Clarke. Cells of the accessory cuneate nucleus give rise to the posterior spinocerebellar tract. (**Ref. 1, p. 119**)

**17. (A)** Afferent and efferent fibers of the cerebral cortex converge toward the brainstem, forming the corona radiata. When these fibers enter the diencephalon they become the internal capsule, a compact band that separates the thalamus from the globus pallidus. (**Ref. 1, pp. 33–34**)

**18. (D)** Axons in the lateral corticospinal tract would most likely have their cell bodies in the contralateral precentral gyrus. Between 75% and 90% of the fibers in the corticospinal tract decussate at caudal medullary levels and enter the posterior part of the lateral funiculus. (**Ref. 1, pp. 210–211**)

**19. (B)** The medial lemniscus is formed by the decussation of fibers from the nuclei cuneatus and gracilis of the opposite side. These fibers can be followed through the brain stem to their termination in the ventral posterolateral nucleus of the thalamus. The decussation of the medial lemniscus contributes to a portion of the sensory input of half the body in the contralateral cerebral cortex. (Ref.1, pp. 116–119)

20. **(B)** A unilateral section of the lateral spinothalamic tract results in a complete loss of pain and thermal sense on the opposite side of the body. This contralateral loss extends to a level on the segment below that of the lesion, owing to the oblique crossing of the fibers. **(Ref. 1, p. 88)**

21. **(B)** These lower motor neurons are responsible for control of all body movements. Loss of these neurons causes complete flaccid paralysis of the muscle, in which the muscle is limp and uncontracted. **(Ref. 1, pp. 73–74)**

22. **(A)** The ventral lateral nucleus is one of the three lateral nuclei of the thalamus. This nucleus is involved in motor control circuits and receives input fibers from the cerebellum and basal ganglia that project to the motor cortex. **(Ref. 1, p. 266)**

23. **(E)** The dorsomedial nucleus is one of two large association nuclei in the thalamus. It is connected with the prefrontal cortex and is involved with functions of affect and foresight. **(Ref. 1, p. 258)**

24. **(C)** The ventricular fasciculus is an efferent projection from the globus pallidus through the internal capsule to the lateral nuclei of the thalamus. **(Ref. 1, p. 341)**

25. **(A)** Disease of upper and lower motor neurons in the spinal cord results in amyotrophic lateral sclerosis. This is a degenerative disease of unknown cause that is characterized by degeneration of the ventral horn cells and corticospinal tracts. **(Ref. 1, p. 107)**

26. **(A)** The thalamic fasciculus is formed by efferent fibers from the medial segment of the globus pallidus (lenticular fasciculus and ansa lenticularis). The fibers of the thalamic fasciculus terminate in the ventral lateral and ventral anterior nuclei of the thalamus. The red nucleus and dentate nucleus do not project to the thalamic fasciculus. **(Ref. 1, p. 342).**

27. **(C)** Each lateral ventricle communicates with the slitlike, midline third ventricle by two short channels, known as the interventricular foramina of Monroe. (**Ref. 1,** p. 40)

28. **(B)** The anterior cerebral artery is a branch of the internal carotid. It supplies the frontal, parietal, and limbic lobes, as well as the paracentral lobule and cingulate gyrus. It also supplies parts of the caudate nucleus, internal capsule, putamen, and septal nuclei. (**Ref. 1,** pp. 441–443)

29. **(A)** Parasympathetic preganglionic neurons located in the superior salivary nucleus of the pons supply the lacrimal, submandibular, mucous, and sublingual glands. The parotid gland is supplied by parasympathetic preganglionic neurons located in the inferior salivary nucleus of the medulla oblongata. (**Ref. 1,** p. 172)

30. **(E)** The gray matter consists of nerve cells and supportive neuroglial elements. It contains parts of myelinated and nonmyelinated fibers along with their cell bodies and dendrites. Within the gray matter, blood vessels also can be found. Fiber tracts course in white matter. (**Ref. 1,** p. 61)

31. **(C)** A fluent aphasia is the condition whereby the patient can produce spoken words but cannot comprehend whether the speech makes any sense. The area of the brain that controls this function is the left parietal lobe. (**Ref. 1,** p. 429)

32. **(B)** The medial longitudinal fasciculus is located near the floor of the fourth ventricle, and consists of fibers that extend to the midbrain and are involved in vestibular functions and eye movements. All of the remaining structures listed are part of the peripheral and central connections of the cochlear pathway. (**Ref. 1,** pp. 153–156)

33. **(B)** The major ascending tracts of the spinal cord include the anterior spinothalamic tract, spinotectal tract, posterior and anterior spinocerebellar tracts, cunecerebellar tract, and spinoreticular tract. Other ascending tracts that have been described are the spinocortical, spino-olivary, spinovestibular, and spinopontine.

The corticospinal tract is a descending motor system. (**Ref. 1,** pp. 83–94)

34. **(C)** Fibers that cross in the spinal cord in the anterior spinothalamic tract mediate light touch (tactile). Those fibers that cross to the opposite side of the cord in the lateral spinothalamic tract mediate pain and temperature. Muscle tone is a motor function of the descending spinal tracts. (**Ref. 1,** pp. 86–88)

35. **(C)** The motor nucleus of the facial nerve consists of a column of multipolar neuron cells located in the ventrolateral part of the reticular formation of the pons, near its caudal border. The facial root fibers emerge from the brain stem near the caudal border of the pons. (**Ref. 1,** pp. 170–173)

36. **(E)** Spinothalamic fibers cross through several spinal segments in the anterior white commissure. Those fibers that ascend contralaterally in the anterolateral and anterior funiculi form the anterior spinothalamic tract. This tract conveys impulses of light touch to higher centers. (**Ref. 1,** p. 86–88)

37. **(D)** The vestibulospinal tract has its origin from the lateral vestibular nucleus, which receives fibers from the vestibular portion of the vestibulocochlear nerve and from specific portions of the cerebellum. Most cells of the lateral vestibular nucleus help form this tract, which descends uncrossed through the entire length of the anterior periphery of the spinal cord. (**Ref. 1,** p. 100)

38. **(B)** Afferent fibers to the substantia nigra arise primarily from the putamen and caudate nucleus. Most of these strionigral fibers terminate upon cells in the pars reticulata. (**Ref. 1,** p. 217)

39. **(A)** The cerebellum furnishes optimum states of tension for all muscles during activity and rest. Thus it is involved with the coordination of somatic motor activity, the mechanisms that influence and maintain equilibrium, skilled movements, and the regulation of muscle tone (**Ref. 1,** pp. 224–237)

40. **(A)** The ventral portion of the pons or pons proper contains the corticopontine fibers, the corticospinal tracts, and the pontine nuclei. The pontine nuclei consist of numerous groups of small and

medium-sized cells situated between the longitudinal and transverse fibers of the pons. The transverse fibers are axons of the pontine nuclei. The pontine nuclei are continuous with the arcuate nuclei of the medulla oblongata. (**Ref. 1,** pp. 46–48)

41. (**E**) There are four nuclear masses associated with the trigeminal nerve. These are the principal sensory nuclei for pressure and tactile sense; the mesencephalic nucleus for proprioceptive impulses; the motor nucleus for the muscles of mastication; and the spinal tract, which relays general somatic afferent fibers through the facial, glossopharyngeal, and vagus nerves. (**Ref. 1,** pp. 178–179)

42. (**B**) The basal ganglia are large nuclear masses that lie in close relationship to the diencephalon but are separated from it by the internal capsule. The basal ganglia include the globus pallidus, caudate nucleus, putamen, subthalamic nucleus, and substantia nigra. (**Ref. 1,** pp. 37–40)

43. (**B**) The central processes of the vestibular afferent fibers enter the brainstem at the pontomedullary junction. These fibers pass through the juxtarestiform body and end mainly in the flocculus and nodulus. (**Ref. 1,** pp. 163–165)

44. (**D**) The ganglionic cell layer is one of the deepest layers of the retina. It comprises the cell bodies of neurons whose axons leave the eye as the optic nerve. These axons converge toward the optic disk, where they form the optic nerve. (**Ref. 1,** pp. 282–284)

45. (**E**) The olfactory tract diverges at the junction between the orbital frontal cortex and anterior perforated substance to form the olfactory trigone. From the trigone, most fibers enter the lateral olfactory stria which is then the principal central pathway to the olfactory cortex for the olfactory system. (**Ref. 1,** pp. 28, 365)

46. (**C**) The diencephalon is subdivided into four major portions: the thalamus, hypothalamus, subthalamus, and epithalamus. The epithalamus consists of stria medullaris, pineal body, habenular trigone, and epithelial portion of the roof of the third ventricle. (**Ref. 1,** pp. 251–255)

**47. (D)** The hypothalamus consists of the ventral walls of the third ventricle inferior to the hypothalamic sulci. It also consists of the structures forming the floor of the ventricle, ie, the tuber cinereum, with the infundibulum, mammillary bodies, optic chiasm, and neurohypophysis. (**Ref. 1,** pp. 317–321)

**48. (A)** The hypothalamus is involved in all types of visceral activities. Lesions of the hypothalamus produce diverse disturbances in autonomic functions including internal secretion, fat and sugar metabolism, eating, water balance, and temperature regulation, and cause somnolence (lethargy and abnormal sleepiness). Dysmetria (overshooting a target) results from lesions of the cerebellum. (**Ref. 1,** pp. 317–321)

**49. (B)** The cerebral hemispheres are joined together by three commissures. The largest and most important of these is the corpus callosum. The anterior commissure and the commissure of the fornix (hippocampal commissure) are the other fiber groups that join the two cerebral hemispheres. (**Ref. 1,** p. 37)

**50. (D)** Various portions of the cerebral cortex within each hemisphere are connected by association fibers. The most prominent of these fibers are the uncinate and arcuate fasciculi and the cingulum. The inferior fibers of the uncinate fasciculus join the posterior orbital gyri with the parahippocampal gyrus. The superior fibers run downward from the frontal to the temporal lobe and connect the orbital gyri of the frontal lobe with the anterior portion of the temporal lobe. (**Ref. 1,** p. 241)

**51. (C)** Relatively little is known about the function of the hippocampus, even though it is a large structure. Available evidence points to the absence of a role for the hippocampus in olfaction. On the other hand, recent studies indicate that the hippocampus may be involved with recent memory. (**Ref. 1,** pp. 375–376)

**52. (E)** The lateral ventricles are found in the cerebral hemispheres and are prolonged by horns into the temporal, parietal, and frontal lobes. The two lateral ventricles are separated by the septum pellucidum. The floor of the lateral ventricles is formed by the caudate nucleus anteriorly and the thalamus posteriorly. (**Ref. 1,** pp. 40–42)

**53. (C)** The medial forebrain bundle consists of fibers that arise from the nasal olfactory regions, periamygdaloid region, and septal nuclei and pass to the lateral portions of the hypothalamus. This bundle joins the ventromedial olfactory centers with the hypothalamus and with the preoptic area rostral and dorsal to the optic chiasm. **(Ref. 1,** p. 304

**54. (D)** The cerebellum receives afferent fibers carrying impulses to it from the cerebrum, mesencephalon, pons, medulla, and spinal cord. From its central nuclei, efferent fibers pass to each of these regions. These connections suggest that the cerebellum serves as an integrative region for the coordination of muscular activity. It has no hypothalamic connections. **(Ref. 1,** pp. 229–232)

**55. (A)** The superior cerebellar peduncle is the most medial and smallest of the three cerebellar peduncles. It is formed from the efferent fibers of the emboliform, globose, and dentate nuclei, which extend to the red nucleus and the thalamus of the opposite side. A number of fibers descend to end in the reticulotegmental nucleus in the upper part of the pons and paramedial reticular nuclei in the medulla. **(Ref. 1,** p. 48)

**56. (C)** The Purkinje cells of the cerebellum are arranged in a single continuous sheet. They are large, flask-shaped cells that are uniformly arranged along the upper edge of the granular layer. Purkinje cells have a darkly staining nucleolus and a clear vesicular cytoplasm. These cells have extensive dendritic ramifications. Their axons are the only ones to enter the white matter of the cerebellar cortex. **(Ref. 1,** p. 227)

**57. (E)** The thalamus is composed primarily of gray matter, within which are the numerous nuclei of this part of the brain. The stratum zonale is a thin layer of white matter on the dorsal surface of the thalamus. Near the internal capsule, along the lateral border of the thalamus, can be seen a band of myelinated fibers that comprises the external medullary lamina. **(Ref. 1,** pp. 255–279)

**58. (B)** The dentate gyrus, part of the archipallium, is like the hippocampus in having three layers: a polymorphic layer, a granular layer, and a molecular layer. The intermediate layer of the hippocampus is called the pyramidal cell layer. **(Ref. 1,** p. 371)

**59. (A)** Two main types of cells are located in the cerebral cortex: the pyramidal cells, which are the most characteristic of the cortex, are the output neurons, while the small, triangular-shaped stellate cells are mainly interneurons. (**Ref. 1,** pp. 390–391)

**60. (B)** The corticobulbar fibers leave the cerebral cortex and descend through the internal capsule to synapse on certain sensory nuclei and some motor nuclei of cranial nerves. These fibers end in the motor nuclei of the trigeminal, facial, and hypoglossal nuclei and the nucleus ambiguus. The Edinger–Westphal nucleus is a column of parasympathetic neurons that project to the ciliary ganglion. (**Ref. 1,** p. 144)

**61. (A)** The giant pyramidal cells are one of the principal types of neurons in the neocortex, and are among the largest neurons in the central nervous system. The axons of these cells leave the cortex and synapse primarily on the alpha motor neurons of the anterior horn of the spinal cord. (**Ref. 1,** pp. 390–393)

**62. (D)** The hypothalamus has connections with the limbic system, pituitary gland, and brain stem, and controls many visceral functions including feeding, drinking, temperature, sexual activity, and gut motility. (**Ref. 1,** p. 303)

**63. (D)** The localized areas to which impulses involved in specific sensory modalities are projected are referred to as the primary sensory areas of the cerebral cortex. The primary sensory areas that have been established for the cerebral cortex are the visual or striate area, auditory area, gustatory area, somesthetic area, and olfactory area. (**Ref. 1,** pp. 401–404)

**64. (A)** The tracts and fibers forming the inferior cerebellar peduncle arise in the spinal cord and medulla. The ascending fibers of this peduncle are primarily the posterior spinocerebellar tract, the crossed olivocerebellar fibers, and the uncrossed accessory cuneate fibers. The remaining tracts are in either the superior or middle cerebellar peduncles. (**Ref. 1,** p. 52)

**65. (E)** The basal ganglia consist of four deeply located masses of gray matter that belong to the cerebral hemispheres or telencephalon. These masses include the amygdaloid, lenticular, and caudate nuclei and the detached portion of the insular cortex called the claustrum. The lenticular and caudate nuclei form the corpus striatum. The globus nucleus is in the cerebellum. (**Ref. 1,** p. 235)

66. **(C)** Two basic types of disturbances are clinically associated with diseases of the basal ganglia. These are abnormal involuntary movements, or dyskinesia, and disturbances related to muscle tone. There are several types of dyskinesia, consisting of tremor, as seen in parkinsonism; athetosis, or slow, writhing involuntary movements, especially of the extremities; chorea, a series of successive involuntary movements; and ballism, a violent flinging movement, especially of the shoulders and pelvic girdles. (**Ref. 1,** pp. 350–353)

67. **(A)** The hippocampus is a long, curved elevation of the temporal lobe that projects into the floor of the inferior horn of the lateral ventricle. It consists of highly specialized cortex of the rhinencephalon. The dentate gyrus, which lies on the medial side of the hippocampus, is separated from the parahippocampal gyrus by the hippocampal fissure. Recent studies indicate that the hippocampus is concerned with recent memory and has no olfactory function. (**Ref. 1,** p. 375)

68. **(D)** The uncus is a short convolution constituting the rostral part of the parahippocampal gyrus that loops around the front end of the hippocampal sulcus. The uncus, anterior part of the parahippocampal gyrus, and lateral olfactory stria form the pyriform lobe. Lesions associated with the uncus may result in olfactory hallucinations or "uncinate fits," which are preceded by disagreeable olfactory sensations. (**Ref. 1,** p. 35)

69. **(E)** The temporal lobes of the cerebrum contain the primary auditory area, gustatory area, and olfactory area. The gustatory area has not been definitely established, but evidence indicates that the sensation for taste is in the parietal operculum and nearby parainsular cortex. The temporal lobes are also involved with memory recall. Visual impulses are associated with the occipital lobes. (**Ref. 1,** p. 27)

**70. (C)** The mesencephalic nucleus of the trigeminal nerve conveys proprioceptive impulses of pressure and kinesthesis from the muscles of mastication, teeth, periodontium, joint capsules, and hard palate. **(Ref. 1, pp. 178–179)**

**71. (A)** The nucleus ambiguus is a group of cells found in the reticular formation. Rostral parts of this cell column give origin to the special visceral efferent fibers that innervate the stylopharyngeus muscle. Fibers from the nucleus ambiguus join efferent fibers from the dorsal motor nucleus of the vagus nerve. **(Ref. 1, p. 141)**

**72. (B)** The hypoglossal nerve innervates the skeletal muscle of the tongue. The nucleus of this nerve forms a column of multipolar motor cells located in the central gray of the medial eminence in the midline of the floor of the fourth ventricle. The root fibers of the nucleus form a series of rootlets that emerge on the surface of the medulla between the pyramid and inferior olivary complex. **(Ref. 1, p. 46)**

**73. (E)** The oculomotor nuclear complex consists of cell columns and nuclei within the mesencephalon that innervate all of the extraocular muscles except the lateral rectus and superior oblique. The complex also supplies the constrictor pupillae muscle. The lateral somatic cell columns innervate the extraocular muscle. The dorsal cell column of the complex innervates the inferior rectus muscle. **(Ref. 1, pp. 203–204)**

**74. (C)** The facial nerve conveys special visceral efferent fibers to branchiomeric muscles derived from the second branchial arch. It also conveys impulses for taste, through the chorda tympani nerve, from the taste buds on the anterior two-thirds of the tongue. **(Ref. 1, pp. 142–144)**

**75. (F)** The hypoglossal nerve begins in the hypoglossal nucleus in the floor of the fourth ventricle of the medulla. Its fibers course along the lateral margin of the medial lemniscus and emerge between the pyramid and inferior olivary. This nerve carries general somatic efferent fibers to the skeletal muscles of the tongue. **(Ref. 1, p. 136)**

76. **(C)** The inferior vestibular nucleus is one of a group of four vestibular nuclei located in the floor of the fourth ventricle. Afferent central fibers from the vestibular ganglion course through the vestibular nerve and synapse in the vestibular nuclei. **(Ref. 1, pp. 161–162)**

77. **(D)** The inferior cerebellar peduncle largely contains afferent fibers from the lateral cuneate nucleus (cuneocerebellar tract) that terminate ipsilaterally in the vermis of the cerebellum. **(Ref. 1, p. 46)**

78. **(G)** The pyramid consists of fibers of the corticospinal descending tract. Most of these fibers (85%) decussate to the contralateral anterior horn cells of the spinal cord. **(Ref. 1, pp. 92, 94–96)**

79. **(A)** The inferior olivary nucleus receives most of its afferent fibers from the ipsilateral red nucleus. Other fibers are derived from the cerebral cortex and spinal cord. Efferent fibers from the olivary nucleus pass through the contralateral inferior cerebellar peduncle to reach the cerebellar cortex. **(Ref. 1, p. 143)**

80. **(B)** The nucleus ambiguus is located in the medullary reticular formation, dorsal to the inferior olivary nucleus. The efferent neurons originating in this nucleus course in cranial nerves IX and X to innervate the muscles of the pharynx. **(Ref. 1, p. 144)**

81. **(E)** The spinal trigeminal nucleus and tract receive and conduct the afferent fibers of the ophthalmic, maxillary, and mandibular divisions of the trigeminal nerve. **(Ref. 1, pp. 177–178)**

82. **(G)** The red nucleus is located in the midbrain tegmentum. All cerebellar projections from this nucleus undergo complete decussation in the midbrain, and the cerveral (corticorubral) projections are partly contralateral and ipsilateral. **(Ref.1, pp. 210–211)**

83. **(B)** The corpus collosum is a large bundle of commissural nerve fibers that extend across the midline, connecting symmetrical areas of the two cerebral hemispheres. It is important in memory and learned discrimination. **(Ref. 1, pp. 37, 393).**

**84. (J)** Posteromedial branches of the posterior cerebral anteries perforate into the medial and anterior parts of the thalamus. Posterior cerebral branches course adjacent to the third ventricle, where they supply the choroid plexus. **(Ref. 1,** pp. 445–448)

**85. (I)** The basal ganglia are subcortical nuclear masses that project to the cerebral motor coxtex. Damage to these nuclei can decrease the ability to control muscular movements. **(Ref. 1,** pp. 350–353)

**86. (F)** The substantia nigra is a large motor nucleus connected to the cerebral cortex, basal ganglia, and hypothalamus. It is involved in muscle tone. **(Ref. 1,** pp. 215–221)

**87. (B)** Tabes dorsalis is a form of neurosyphilis and is characterized by degeneration in the dorsal roots, posterior columns, and pretectal region (mesencephalon). **(Ref. 1,** p. 112)

**88. (E)** Argyll–Robertson pupils occur with lesions of the pretectal region near the cerebral aqueduct, and are characterized by loss or diminution of pupillary constriction in the pupillary light reflex, while the pupillary constriction of the accommodation reflex remains intact. The afferent limb of the accommodation reflex is volitional (cortically engendered) and is not transmitted through pretectal neurons to the Edinger–Westphal nucleus. The pupillary light reflex is produced by light stimuli transmitted via the optic nerve to pretectal neurons and then to the nucleus of Edinger–Westphal. **(Ref. 1,** pp. 205–206)

**89. (C)** Romberg's sign, in which the patient tends to sway or fall when standing with the feet together and eyes closed, indicates damage to the integrity of the posterior columns. The eyes must be closed to elicit the sign, since vision can, in part, substitute for proprioception (position sense). **(Ref. 1,** pp. 116–119)

**90. (B)** Ataxia occurred in this patient when degeneration in the posterior columns interfered with the transmission of proprioceptive and vibratory sense information into the central nervous system. When this happens, the motor performance of gait cannot cannot be controlled. **(Ref. 1,** p. 245)

**91. (D)** Areflexia occurred in this patient when degeneration in the posterior columns interfered with the transmission of proprioceptive and vibratory sense information into the central nervous system. When this happens, the sensory limb of reflex arcs is lost. **(Ref. 1,** p. 117)

**92. (A)** Weber's syndrome (superior alternating hemiplegia) is characterized by ipsilateral oculomotor nerve (lower motor neurons) involvement and damage to the contralateral corticospinal tract (upper motor neurons). **(Ref. 1,** p. 210)

**93. (D)** The oculomotor nerve passes through and around the pes pedunculi, which contains axons of the corticospinal and corticobulbar tracts. Emerging in the interpeduncular fosa, the oculomotor nerve grooves the medial side of the pes, lying between the posterior cerebral and superior cerebellar arteries. **(Ref. 1,** pp. 203–204)

**94. (C)** The portion of the facial nucleus controlling the upper face muscles receives bilateral projections from the corticobulbar tract, while the portion controlling the lower facial muscles receives only contralateral projections. In upper motor neuron damage, the tip of the tongue turns to the side opposite the lesion. In this case the lesion is on the left, so the tip of the tongue turns to the right. The genioglossus muscle protrudes the tongue. Neurons of the hypoglossal nucleus that innervate the genioglossus muscle convey only contralateral corticobulbar control. The imbalance in function of the two sides of the tongue, when protruded, results in the left side of the forward thrust of the tongue being unopposed because the paralyzed right side lags behind. Consequently, the tip of the tongue turns to the right. **(Ref. 1,** pp. 144–146)

**95. (E)** Extension of the great toe and fanning of the four lateral toes following a stroking stimulus to the sole of the foot suggests damage to the contralateral corticospinal tract. In the intact adult, the normal response to the stimulus is flexion and adduction of the toes. **(Ref. 1,** pp. 107–111)

**96. (B)** Damage to the corticospinal tract results in hypertonia, hyperreflexia, spastic paralysis, loss of superficial reflexes, and the Babinski sign. **(Ref. 1,** pp. 107–108, 421–423)

**97. (C)** The oculomotor nerve innervates the levator palpebrae superioris muscle, which elevates the upper eyelid. The parasympathetic component of the nerve innervates the smooth muscle that constricts the pupil as well as the ciliary muscle, which controls lens diameter. (**Ref. 1,** pp. 203–204)

**98. (D)** The structures involved in the lesion are in the dorsolateral medulla, including the nucleus ambiguus (cranial nerves IX and X), inferior cerebellar peduncle, vestibular nuclei, spinal trigeminal tract, lateral spinothalamic tract, and descending hypothalamic axons in the dorsolateral tegmentum. (**Ref. 1,** pp. 192, 210)

**99. (B)** Wallenberg's syndrome is the eponym for the dorsolateral medullary syndrome. (**Ref. 1,** pp. 121, 148)

**100. (E)** Hypotonia and hyporeflexia are characteristic of cerebellar involvement and result in ataxia. This is probably caused by interruption of some cerebellar afferents via the inferior cerebellar peduncle. Vertigo with falling to the right indicates involvement of vestibular nuclei or their afferents to the cerebellum. (**Ref. 1,** pp. 245–246)

**101. (C)** The slight ptosis of Horner's syndrome is caused by dysfunction of the smooth muscle of the upper eyelid, Muller's tarsal muscle. (**Ref. 1,** p. 210)

**102. (A)** Axons of hypothalamic nuclei descending in the brain stem to reach the lower motor neurons (intermediolateral cell column) direct the sympathetic visceral function of smooth muscle, cardiac muscle, and glands throughout the body. (**Ref. 1,** pp. 298–203)

**103. (C)** Sensations of pain and temperature are transmitted from the left side of the body below the head by the lateral spinothalamic tract, which lies in the right lateral medulla, since the tract crosses at spinal levels. However, the right spinal trigeminal tract, transmitting pain and temperature sensation from the right side of the face, is ipsilateral. (**Ref. 1,** pp. 88, 129)

**104. (B)** Muller's tarsal muscle is smooth muscle receiving sympathetic innervation via the internal carotid plexus. **(Ref. 1,** pp. 438–449)

**105. (E)** Bulbar branches of the vertebral artery and posterior inferior cerebellar artery supply the dorsolateral medulla. The distribution of the posterior inferior cerebellar artery is the more extensive of the two. **(Ref. 1,** pp. 434, 449–455)

**106. (B)** The mental symptoms in this case suggest Korsakoff's syndrome, with lesions involving the hypothalamus, especially the mammillary bodies. **(Ref. 1,** p. 375)

**107. (E)** Polyneuritis results from degeneration of the peripheral nerves with associated pain, paresthesias, and some sensory loss. **(Ref. 1,** p. 107)

**108. (A)** The term "limbic system" includes those structures that are part of the limbic lobe, as well as subcortical nuclei and major connecting bundles. These are located in an area extending from the septal area to the mesencephalic tegmentum. The cerebellar peduncles are not known to carry projections of the limbic system. **(Ref. 1,** pp. 384–386)

**109. (D)** Poor nutrition and vitamin deficiency, especially thiamine deficiency, are believed to be the cause of Korsakoff's syndrome. **(Ref. 1,** pp. 245–246)

**110. (C)** The limbic lobe forms a limbus, or halo, about the diencephalon. The mammillary bodies are hypothalamic nuclei. **(Ref. 1,** pp. 31–32)

**111. (B)** Lesions in the mammillary bodies are seen in Korsakoff's syndrome and often in the medial dorsal thalamic nucleus as well. **(Ref. 1,** pp. 302–303)

**112. (B)** Pill-rolling tremor, tremor at rest, poverty of movement, and lack of facial expression are all signs of Parkinson's disease (paralysis agitans). **(Ref. 1,** p. 351)

**113. (C)** Depletion of dopamine in nigral neurons occurs in Parkinson's disease. (**Ref. 1,** pp. 215–221).

**114. (E)** Neurons of the substantia nigra form dopamine. (**Ref. 1,** pp. 216–217)

**115. (A)** Dopaminergic neurons in the substantia nigra project to the corpus striatum and release dopamine at their terminals. (**Ref. 1,** p. 217)

**116. (B)** Because dopamine does not cross the blood–brain barrier, a dopamine precursor, L-dihydroxyphenylalanine (L-dopa), is used in treating Parkinson's disease. (**Ref. 1,** pp. 353–354)

**117. (E)** The right internal strabismus occurs because the right lateral rectus muscle, innervated by the right abducens nerve, cannot function. The right eye remains swung medially because of the unopposed pull. (**Ref. 1,** pp. 174–175)

**118. (B)** The signs of upper motor neuron damage are on the left because, in a pontine lesion, the right corticospinal tract has not yet crossed. (**Ref. 1,** pp. 94–96)

**119. (D)** Middle alternating hemiplegia is characterized by ipsilateral damage to the abducens nerve (lower motor neurons) and contralateral damage to the corticospinal tract (upper motor neurons). (**Ref. 1,** p. 174)

**120. (B)** The abducens nerve exits the basilar pons through axons of the adjacent cortocospinal tract, which has not yet crossed. (**Ref. 1,** p. 174–175)

**121. (A)** The extrapyramidal motor system sets a pattern of gross postural movement upon which the more discrete skilled movement engineered by the corticospinal tract is imposed. When the corticospinal tract is damaged, the movement mediated by the extrapyramidal system can become apparent. (**Ref. 1,** p. 95)

**122. (C)** Paramedian branches of the basilar artery directly penetrate the basilar pons. (**Ref. 1,** p. 449)

**123. (B)**   The only circumscribed site in the central nervous system at which such extensive motor and sensory loss can follow a single lesion is the posterior limb of the internal capsule, in this case the right posterior limb. (**Ref. 1,** pp. 279–283)

**124. (D)**   Sweeping from the lateral geniculate body to project posteriorly, the geniculocalcarine tract is immediately in a retrolenticular position. (**Ref. 1,** pp. 250, 283)

**125. (A)**   The superior thalamic peduncle of the posterior limb contains the final thalamocortical projection of the pain, temperature, and proprioceptive pathways, as well as the corticospinal tract. (**Ref. 1,** p. 280)

**126. (E)**   Fibers of the auditory radiation sweep inferiorly to the posterior limb and lenticular nucleus to reach the transverse temporal gyri. (**Ref. 1,** pp. 156–159)

**127. (D)**   The anterior choroidal artery, branching from the internal carotid artery, supplies a large part of the posterior limb and all of the retrolenticular part. The lateral striate arteries, branches of the middle cerebral artery, also contribute to the posterior limb. (**Ref. 1,** p. 283)

**128. (C)**   Descent of corticospinal tract axons in the posterior limb places them in a small area with the great sensory systems. (**Ref. 1,** p. 282)

**129. (L)**   The dentate gyrus is the inner layer of the hippocampal formation. It consists of three layers that give rise to fibers extending into the hippocampal formation. Recent evidence suggest the lesions of he hippocampus and dentate gyrus result in significant loss of recent memory with mild behavorial changes. (**Ref. 1,** pp. 371, 375)

**130. (H)**   The locus ceruleus is a collection of heavily pigmented cells in the periventricular gray, adjacent to the fourth ventricle and consisting of norepinephrine-containing neurons. The efferent projections of the locus ceruleus play a prominent role in paradoxical sleep and inhibition of sensory neurons. (**Ref. 1,** p. 184)

**131. (P)**   Many of the afferent fibers to the rostral part of the red nucleus are derived from the dentate nucleus of the opposite side. This nucleus is the largest of the deep cerebellar nuclei in the white matter of the cerebellum. (**Ref. 1,** p. 210)

**132. (N)**   Injuries to different parts of the optic pathway will produce visual defects based on their location. Lesions of the temporal lobe destroy the looping fibers in the inferior optic radiation, resulting in homonymous quadrantic defects. (**Ref. 1,** pp. 287–288)

**133. (A)**   The lateral lemniscus is a definitive bundle of fibers located near the lateral surface of the tegmentum. It is the main ascending auditory pathway in the brain stem. (**Ref. 1,** p. 157)

**134. (G)**   The pineal body contains a network of vascular connective tissue comprising glial cells and pinealocytes. The latter cells are secretary and produce serotonin, norepinephrine, and melatonin. (**Ref. 1,** p. 253)

**135. (E)**   The pars triangularis and pars opercularis are located in the dominant inferior fontal gyrus, and are called the Broca's speech area. Lesions in this area produce a motor speech apraxia. (**Ref. 1,** p. 26)

# 3

# Microanatomy

---

**DIRECTIONS (Questions 1–184):** Each of the questions or incomplete statements below is followed by five suggested answers or completions. Select the **one** that is best in each case.

---

1. Which of the following cells in the central nervous system is homologous to the Schwann cell of the peripheral nervous system?
   A. astrocyte
   B. satellite cell
   C. protoplasmic astrocyte
   D. oligodendrocyte
   E. fibrous astrocyte

2. During the proliferative (follicular) phase of the menstrual cycle, one can observe that
   A. the endometrium thickens largely because of edema
   B. glycogen disappears in the basal cytoplasm of the glandular epithelium
   C. there is a two-to-threefold increase in the thickness of the endometrium
   D. the endometrial glands become quite tortuous
   E. blood pours into the stroma and soon breaks into the uterine lumen

3. The cell organelle that is responsible for phosphorylation is the
   A. smooth endoplasmic reticulum
   B. mitochondria
   C. nucleolus
   D. rough endoplasmic reticulum
   E. Golgi apparatus

4. The structural unit of collagen, tropocollagen, is synthesized by
   A. macrophages
   B. fibroblasts
   C. megakaryoctyes
   D. plasma cells
   E. monocytes

5. The function of the interstitial endocrine cells of the testis is to
   A. form the acrosome
   B. secrete testosterone
   C. support the germinal epithelium
   D. supply nutrients to the sex cells
   E. inhibit spermatogenesis

6. Which part of the skeletal muscle fiber is most closely associated with adenosine triphosphatase (ATPase) activity?
   A. actin
   B. T tubule
   C. sarcotubules
   D. light meromysin
   E. heavy meromysin

7. The organelles that supply energy for numerous cell reactions are the
   A. lysosomes
   B. centrioles
   C. Golgi apparatus
   D. mitochondria
   E. ribosomes

8. The cell organelles that play an important role in the intracellular digestion of phagocytosed particles are called
   A. the Golgi apparatus
   B. lysosomes
   C. ribosomes
   D. centrosomes
   E. mitochondria

9. The Golgi apparatus has been shown to be a site for the
   A. concentration of secretory products
   B. synthesis of protein
   C. production of enzymes
   D. production of acid hydrolases
   E. intracellular digestion of degradation products

10. The respiratory bronchiole differs from the terminal bronchiole in that the former
    A. lacks cilia
    B. contains goblet cells
    C. has a small amount of cartilage
    D. is lined by ciliated columnar epithelium
    E. contains a few alveoli

11. In the central nervous system, macrophages are formed by
    A. astrocytes
    B. oligodendroglia
    C. microglia
    D. ependyma
    E. satellite cells

12. During intramembranous ossification, ossification first begins in
    A. cartilage
    B. bone
    C. mesenchyme
    D. dense irregular connective tissue
    E. calcified cartilage matrix

13. Myelin is formed by
    A. Schwann cells
    B. satellite cells
    C. ependyma

D. astrocytes
E. microglia

14. The granules found in the cells of the adrenal medulla consist of
    A. hydrocortisone
    B. glucocorticoids
    C. epinephrine
    D. mineralocorticoids
    E. androgens

15. The tunica vasculosa (uvea) of the eye comprises each of the following **EXCEPT** the
    A. ciliary body
    B. iris
    C. choroid
    D. sclera
    E. ciliary muscle

16. Synapses may be clasified on the basis of each of the following **EXCEPT**
    A. position
    B. membrane specialization
    C. organelle content
    D. synaptic vesicle content
    E. shape of end bulb

17. Which of the following is a nonencapsulated afferent nerve ending?
    A. pacinian corpuscle
    B. Kraus end bulb
    C. Meissner corpuscle
    D. Merkel ending
    E. Ruffini corpuscle

18. Which of the following characterizes the secretory stage of the menstrual cycle?
    A. the endomentrium hypertrophies due to hypertrophy of the gland cells
    B. ripening of ovarian follicles
    C. rapid regeneration of the endometrium
    D. glands become tortuous
    E. coiled arteries make their appearance

**19.** The morphologic changes associated with skeletal muscle contraction include each of the following **EXCEPT**
   A. the muscle fiber becomes shorter and broader
   B. each sarcomere becomes shorter
   C. absence of adenosine triphosphate (ATP) release
   D. the I band becomes shorter and eventually disappears at 50% contraction
   E. the total length of the A band remains constant

**20.** Each of the following characterizes the female urethra **EXCEPT**
   A. it has mucosal glands
   B. it is usually lined with stratified squamous epithelium
   C. its lamina propria is thin and contains smooth muscle
   D. it has a sphincter urethrae consisting of skeletal muscle
   E. its muscular coat contains two layers of smooth muscle

**21.** Each of the following is associated with the ductus deferens **EXCEPT**
   A. it has stereocilia
   B. its muscular coat consists of two layers
   C. it is lined by pseudostratified columnar epithelium
   D. it has a lumen with a highly irregular outline because of folds in the epithelium and lamina propria
   E. it conducts sperm

**22.** Each of the following characterizes the rod cells of the human retina **EXCEPT**
   A. they are important in night vision
   B. they are least numerous in the region of the fovea centralis
   C. they contain a pigment known as rhodopsin
   D. they are important in color vision
   E. they are taller than cone cells

**23.** Deoxyribunucleic acid (DNA) is found only in the
   A. nucleus
   B. mitochondria
   C. golgi apparatus
   D. lysosomes
   E. ribosomes

24. Adhering to the outer surface of the limiting membrane of the granular endoplasmic reticulum are
    A. mitochondria
    B. lysosomes
    C. ribosomes
    D. Golgi particles
    E. vacuoles

25. Chromatids are formed during
    A. interphase
    B. prophase
    C. metaphase
    D. telophase
    E. anaphase

26. One type of epithelium may change into another by a process called
    A. regeneration
    B. amitosis
    C. meiosis
    D. pinocytosis
    E. metaplasia

27. Simple cuboidal epithelium is usually found in
    A. the inner surface of the tympanic membrane of the ear
    B. the parietal layer of Bowman's capsule
    C. the descending limb of the loop of Henle
    D. the rete testis
    E. a single layer on the free surface of the ovary

28. The cells lining the ventricles of the brain and central canal of the spinal cord are known as
    A. astrocytes
    B. microglia
    C. oligodendroglia
    D. ependymal cells
    E. satellite cells

**29.** Erythrocytes are characterized by each of the following **EXCEPT**
  **A.** they are nonmotile
  **B.** they lack a nucleus
  **C.** they are devoid of mitochondria
  **D.** they are pale, greenish yellow
  **E.** they do not function in carrying oxygen

**30.** Types of neuroglia include each of the following **EXCEPT**
  **A.** astrocytes
  **B.** microglia
  **C.** plasmacytes
  **D.** ependymal cells
  **E.** oligodendrocytes

**31.** In large elastic arteries, each of the following is correct **EXCEPT**
  **A.** there is a thin basement membrane
  **B.** the endothelium is composed of a single layer of cells
  **C.** the tunica media consists largely of elastic tissue
  **D.** the tunica adventitia is thin
  **E.** the walls may contain smooth muscle fibers

**32.** Sinusoids are correctly described by each of the following **EXCEPT**
  **A.** they have a irregular, tortuous lumen
  **B.** they are lined by endothelial cells
  **C.** they have a dense connective tissue wall
  **D.** they have a limited disrtibution in some organs
  **E.** they have no phagocytic elements

**33.** The thymus is described by each of the following **EXCEPT**
  **A.** the medulla contains reticular cells
  **B.** the medulla contains Hassal bodies
  **C.** the medulla is more vascular than the cortex
  **D.** cells similar to lymphocytes are present in the cortex
  **E.** it has no efferent lymphatics

**34.** The parotid gland is characterized by
  **A.** being entirely serous
  **B.** containing secretory granules
  **C.** being a compound tubuloalveolar gland

   **D.** having a definite capsule
   **E.** having many intralobular ducts

**35.** During contraction of skeletal muscle, calcium is released from the
   **A.** transverse (T) tubules
   **B.** sarcoplasmic reticulum
   **C.** Golgi apparatus
   **D.** scarcoplasm
   **E.** A bands

**36.** The Nissl bodies located in the cell bodies of motor neurons are formed by
   **A.** mitochondria
   **B.** nuclei
   **C.** dendrites
   **D.** microtubules
   **E.** rough endoplasmic reticulum

**37.** Which of the following types of cells constitutes the defense against invasion of bacteria and other microorganisms?
   **A.** erythrocytes
   **B.** platelets
   **C.** neutrophils
   **D.** lymphocytes
   **E.** basophils

**38.** An identifying feature of the esophagus is
   **A.** a presence of glands
   **B.** a tube consisting mainly of connective tissue
   **C.** epithelium of simple columnar type
   **D.** a lamina propria of dense connective tissue
   **E.** the absence of a tunica adventitia

**39.** Regulation of the size of the lumen of bronchioles is controlled by
   **A.** collagen
   **B.** smooth muscle and elastic fibers
   **C.** cartilage
   **D.** elastic fibers and cartilage
   **E.** pseudostratified ciliated columnar epithelium

**40.** The pars distalis of the pituitary gland contains
   A. pituicytes
   B. pinealocytes
   C. acidophils and basophils
   D. axons of neurons of the paraventricular nucleus
   E. cells that secrete parathormone

**41.** The function of the parathyroid glands is to
   A. produce thryrocalcitonin
   B. produce a hormone that raises blood glucose
   C. produce a hormone that regulates blood calcium levels
   D. secrete albumin
   E. function antagonistically to the adrenal gland

**42.** Cells in the epidermis that contain tyrosinase are
   A. known as Langerhan cells
   B. involved in the production of melanin
   C. known as Merkel cells
   D. touch receptors
   E. actually bipolar neurons

**43.** The subcapsular (marginal) sinus of lymph nodes would normally contain all the following **EXCEPT**
   A. reticular cells
   B. reticular fibers
   C. macrophages
   D. erythrocytes
   E. lymphocytes

**44.** Each of the following statements concerning the interstitial cells of Leydig is true **EXCEPT** that they
   A. are located in the angular spaces among seminiferous tubules
   B. have much smooth endoplasmic reticulum
   C. secrete testosterone
   D. are controlled by hypophyseal follicle-stimulating hormone (FSH)
   E. contain cytoplasmic granules of Reinke

**45.** Semen is composed of products produced by all of the following **EXCEPT** the
   A. prostate gland
   B. seminiferous tubules
   C. bulbourethral glands
   D. rete testis
   E. seminal vesicles

**46.** Bile formed by hepatic cells is first secreted into the
   A. bile canaliculi
   B. space of Disse
   C. bile ducts
   D. ampulla of Vater
   E. hepatic duct

**47.** The glands of Von Ebner are characteristic of the
   A. pyloroduodenal junction
   B. lamina propria of the esophagus
   C. circumvallate papillae
   D. oral mucosa of the lip
   E. intestinal villi

**48.** The periosteum is firmly attached to compact bone by
   A. processes from endosteal osteocytes
   B. fibers from Voilkmann's canals
   C. outer circumferential lamellae
   D. Sharpey's fibers
   E. fibers from interstitial lamellae

**49.** Premature infants who exhibit the respiratory distress syndrome have an absence of
   A. goblet cells
   B. type I alveolar cells
   C. dust cells
   D. type II alveolar cells
   E. Clara cells

**50.** Expiration of air from the pulmonary alveoli occurs as a result of
   A. smooth muscle in the terminal bronchioles
   B. elastic recoil in the alveolar walls
   C. expansion of the rib cage
   D. negative pressure in the pleural cavity
   E. innervation of the bronchi

**51.** The cortical labyrinth of the kidney contains
   A. thin segments of Henle's loop
   B. proximal convoluted tubules
   C. renal columns
   D. papillary ducts
   E. the peritubular vascular plexus

**52.** Both skeletal and smooth muscle can be found in the muscularis externa of the
   A. stomach
   B. duodenum
   C. colon
   D. jejunum
   E. esophagus

**53.** According to the "closed" theory of circulation within the spleen, blood leaving the terminal capillaries enters directly into
   A. splenic sinuses
   B. pulp veins
   C. pulp (Billroth's) cords
   D. penicilli
   E. trabecular veins

**54.** A principal difference between spongy and compact bone is the
   A. composition of the amorphous ground substance
   B. amount of collagen in the matrix
   C. presence or absence of osseous lamellae
   D. manner in which they arise; one is by endochondral and the other by intramembranous ossification
   E. ratio of bone matrix to soft tissue spaces

**55.** A purely serous gland possessing no striated ducts but having long intercalated ducts and centroacinar cells is the
   A. submandibular gland
   B. pancreas
   C. sublingual gland
   D. parotid gland
   E. Brunner's gland

**56.** The chief cells of the stomach are more numerous in
   A. the base region of gastric (zymogenic) glands in the fundus
   B. gastric pits of gastric glands
   C. the base region of pyloric gastric glands
   D. the isthmus region of cardiac gastric glands
   E. the neck region of gastric glands in the fundus

**57.** The following secretions are correctly matched with their cells of origin in every pair **EXCEPT**
   A. glucagon–pancreatic alpha cells
   B. intrinsic factor–parietal cells of the stomach
   C. insulin–pancreatic beta cells
   D. hydrochloric acid–chief cells of the stomach
   E. mucus–Brunner's glands

**58.** All of the following are correct concerning the male reproductive system **EXCEPT**
   A. the ductus deferens is lined by pseudostratified columnar epithelium
   B. the ejaculatory duct epithelium may be simple or pseudostratified columnar
   C. the motile cilia of the ductus deferens epithelium sweep mature sperm toward the ejaculatory ducts
   D. the prostate is a compund tubuloalveolar gland
   E. crystalloids of Reinke may be found in the cytoplasm of Leydig cells

**59.** In the mature sperm each of the following is correct **EXCEPT**
   A. the acrosomal material is derived from the Golgi complex
   B. a typical 9+2 microtuble assembly is present in the flagellum
   C. a haploid number of chromosomes is present
   D. the mitochondrial sheath is found in the middle piece
   E. motility is dependent on the total number of spermatozoa

**60.** Which is the best set of characteristics you can use to distinguish the three muscle cell types from each other?
  **A.** cell shape and nuclear shape
  **B.** cell shape, nuclear position, and number
  **C.** cell shape and presence of intercalated discs
  **D.** nuclear shape and presence of sarcomeres
  **E.** striations

**61.** The neuromusclar junction is a specialized form of synaptic contact between motoneuron axon terminals and muscle. Which of the following properties distinguishes it from a central nervous system synapse?
  **A.** the presence of junctional folds of the postsynaptic membrane
  **B.** the presence of synaptic vesicles within the presynaptic axon
  **C.** the presence of a postsynaptic receptor membrane
  **D.** the presence of a synaptic cleft
  **E.** the presence of presynaptic membrane specialization

**62.** Keratohyalin granules of skin are characteristically present in the
  **A.** stratum corneum
  **B.** stratum spinosum
  **C.** stratum granulosum
  **D.** stratum germinativum
  **E.** stratum lucidum

**63.** Sebaceous and sweat glands are similar in that
  **A.** they are both extensions of the epidermis
  **B.** they secrete the same substances
  **C.** they are both connected to the hair follicle
  **D.** their modes of secretion are identical
  **E.** they are both simple coiled tubular glands

**64.** The glomerulus of the renal corpuscle has which of the following two blood vessels associated with it?
  **A.** an artery and a vein
  **B.** an afferent and an efferent vein
  **C.** a glomerular artery and a glomerular vein
  **D.** an afferent and an efferent arteriole
  **E.** two capillaries

**65.** The urinary bladder is lined with
   **A.** stratified squamous epithelium
   **B.** transitional epithelium
   **C.** pseudostratified squamous epithelium
   **D.** simple squamous epithelium
   **E.** cuboidal epithelium

**66.** The vagina and esophagus are similar in that both have
   **A.** a muscularis mucosa
   **B.** glands in the lamina propria
   **C.** scattered skeletal muscle fibers in the muscularis externa
   **D.** a stratified squamous epithelium
   **E.** no muscularis mucosa

**67.** Which of the following epithelia can usually be found in the normal female reproductive tract?
   **A.** stratified squamous and simple columnar
   **B.** transitional and stratified squamous
   **C.** simple columnar and transitional
   **D.** simple columnar and pseudostratified
   **E.** pseudostratified

**68.** Ovarian follicle cells contribute to the following **EXCEPT**
   **A.** corpus luteum
   **B.** zona pellucida
   **C.** production of luteinizing hormone
   **D.** granulosa cells
   **E.** theca cells

**69.** A corpus albicans
   **A.** secretes estrogen
   **B.** is actually a degenerated corpus luteum
   **C.** secretes progesterone
   **D.** is never found before or after puberty
   **E.** forms the ovarian follicle

**70.** Growth of hyaline cartilage
   A. is rapid and requires good vascularization
   B. requires chondrocytes and chondroclasts
   C. requires a perichondrium to give rise to chondrocytes
   D. does not form a matrix
   E. may be intramembranous or endochondral

**71.** A portal triad includes a branch of each of the following **EXCEPT** the
   A. portal vein
   B. hepatic artery
   C. bile duct
   D. central vein
   E. lymphatics

**72.** In the kidney, one would expect to find glomeruli almost exclusively confined to the
   A. cortex
   B. renal pelvis
   C. medulla
   D. capsule
   E. loop of Henle

**73.** Two sets of overlapping thick and thin filaments occur in the myofibril. In terms of their protein content they mainly contain
   A. troponin and actin
   B. myosin and actin
   C. troponin and tropomyosin
   D. myosin and troponin
   E. filamin and tropomyosin

**74.** The most important factor in transporting sperm through the uterus and oviducts is probably
   A. the direction of fluid flow
   B. positive rheotaxis
   C. flagellations of the sperm tail
   D. beating of cilia of uterine and oviductal epithelium
   E. muscular contractions of the uterus and oviducts

**75.** Phagocytosis is usually associated with
   **A.** erythrocytes
   **B.** mast cells
   **C.** neutrophils
   **D.** basophils
   **E.** plasma cells

**76.** Drug detoxification occurs in the
   **A.** Golgi apparatus
   **B.** smooth endoplasmic reticulum
   **C.** rough endoplasmic reticulum
   **D.** lysosomes
   **E.** nucleus

**77.** A protein secretory cell usually synthesizes protein in which organelle?
   **A.** Golgi apparatus
   **B.** smooth endoplasmic reticulum
   **C.** rough endoplasmic reticulum
   **D.** cytoplasm
   **E.** mitochondrion

**78.** Mitochondrial cristae have the important function of
   **A.** converting adenosine diphosphate (ADP) to adenosine triphosphate (ATP)
   **B.** making protein
   **C.** changing adenosine monophosphate (AMP) to ADP
   **D.** producing lipids, carbohydrates, and amino acids
   **E.** allowing substances to pass because of their extreme permeability

**79.** Lysosomes are important in each of the following **EXCEPT**
   **A.** digestion of phagosome contents
   **B.** macrophages
   **C.** containing hydrolytic enzymes
   **D.** making protein
   **E.** autolysis of the cell

**80.** Stratified squamous keratinizing epithelium is characterized by
 **A.** cells that all are nucleated
 **B.** many nerves
 **C.** many mucus cells
 **D.** many cilia
 **E.** protection of deeper epithelial cells

**81.** The three types of granulocytes usually can be distinguished best under the light microscope on the basis of
 **A.** nuclear morphology and cell size
 **B.** cell size only
 **C.** cell shape only
 **D.** staining reaction of cytoplasmic granules
 **E.** nuclear morphology only

**82.** Platelets
 **A.** have a spherical nucleus
 **B.** release ADP and clotting factors when activated
 **C.** are found in connective tissue
 **D.** are stored in the liver
 **E.** can be increased in number by erythropoietin

**83.** All of the striations observed in skeletal muscle under the light microscope are due to
 **A.** vertical alignment of sarcomeres
 **B.** horizontal alignment of triads
 **C.** myofibrils arranged like collagen to give a similar banding pattern
 **D.** vertical alignment of T-tubules
 **E.** vertical alignment of triads

**84.** The sarcoplasmic reticulum
 **A.** is part of the neuromuscular junction
 **B.** inhibits calcium production
 **C.** is continuous with the T-tubules
 **D.** is more abundant in cardiac than skeletal muscle
 **E.** releases calcium which allows actin to interact with myosin

**85.** Cardiac and skeletal muscle are different in that
   **A.** only skeletal muscle is influenced by nerves
   **B.** only skeletal muscle has intercalated discs
   **C.** only cardiac muscle has inherent rhythmicity
   **D.** only cardiac muscle has transverse striations
   **E.** only skeletal muscle has central nuclei

**86.** Smooth muscle is described by each of the following **EXCEPT**
   **A.** is characterized by thick, thin, and intermediate contractile filaments
   **B.** it has sarcomeres arranged in a manner similar to that of skeletal muscle
   **C.** it can only be stimulated by nerves of the autonomic nervous system
   **D.** its contraction is regulated by concentration of calcium ions
   **E.** it has elongated, tapered cells

**87.** Plasma cells
   **A.** contain few ribosomes
   **B.** have a centrally located nucleus
   **C.** are specialized for the production of humoral antibodies
   **D.** are found mostly in lymphatic tissue
   **E.** are not active in protein secretion

**88.** Tissue macrophages are
   **A.** derived from B-lymphocytes
   **B.** highly phagocytic and rich in lysosomes
   **C.** not part of the reticuloendothelial system
   **D.** mast cells
   **E.** the producers of connective tissue fibers

**89.** The fibrous component of loose connective tissue is composed of
   **A.** collagenous, reticular, and elastic fibers
   **B.** type I collagen in loose bundles
   **C.** elastin, collagen, and glycoproteins
   **D.** type III collagen in fine fibers
   **E.** interstitial collagen

**90.** Collagen is secreted by fibroblasts, smooth muscle cells, and chondroctyes
   A. as microfibrils
   B. within the Golgi apparatus
   C. as quarter-staggered tropocollagen molecules
   D. as reticulin
   E. as procollagen, with nonhelical extensions

**91.** Chondrocytes are nourished by
   A. dissolved nutrients passing through the cartilage matrix
   B. a system of canaliculi between lacunae
   C. the vascular network within the territorial matrix
   D. glycogen and lipid stores
   E. calcified matrix channels

**92.** Cartilage matrix contains type II collagen and
   A. a hydrophilic proteoglycan complex
   B. a hyaluronic acid bound to the collagen
   C. a hyaluronic acid-chondroitin sulfate copolymer
   D. a chondroitin sulfate–proteoglycan complex bound to fibronectin
   E. a hyaluronic acid–unsulfated glycosaminoglycan complex

**93.** Appositional growth of cartilage
   A. produces territorial matrix in apposition to chondroblasts
   B. causes clones of chondroctyes to form
   C. adds matrix but not cells to cartilage
   D. occurs from the chondrogenic layer of the perichondrium
   E. is the differentiation of chondroctyes from mesenchyme

**94.** The two most abundant inorganic components of bone matrix are
   A. calcium carbonate and sodium citrate
   B. magnesium sulfate and calcium sulfate
   C. calcium phosphate and calcium carbonate
   D. calcium fluoride and magnesium carbonate
   E. calcium phosphate and magnesium sulfate

**95.** The Haversian canals of bone tissue
   A. contain chondroctyes
   B. are not common in spongy bone trabeculae

C. form the central structures of a Haversian system
D. are lined by cement lines
E. run perpendicular to the long axis of the bone

96. Reticular cells of epithelial origin are found in
   A. the spleen
   B. the thymus
   C. the tonsil
   D. the lymph nodes
   E. Peyer's patches

97. Regions of lymphatic organs that depend specifically upon the thymus for normal maintainence and function (ie, thymus-dependent regions) include
   A. the cortex of tonsils and medulla of lymph nodes
   B. the paracortical region of lymph nodes and periarterial lymphatic sheaths of the spleen
   C. the deep cortical region and medullary cords of lymph nodes
   D. the medullae of lymph nodes and tonsils
   E. the paracortical region of lymph nodes and the splenic red pulp

98. The vessels whose adventitia is described as having longitudinal bundles of collagen and elastic fibers and isolated longitudinal bundles of smooth muscle are
   A. elastic arteries
   B. muscular arteries
   C. capillaries
   D. large veins
   E. venules

99. Fenestrated capillaries have
   A. extremely attenuated areas of endothelium with pores
   B. thickened areas with pores
   C. a discontinuous basal lamina
   D. diaphragms that have the same thickness as unit membranes
   E. pores that are evenly spaced over the entire surface of the endothelium

**100.** Pancreatic islet beta cells secrete
- **A.** somatostatin
- **B.** insulin
- **C.** glucagon
- **D.** secretin
- **E.** intrinsic factor

**101.** Spermiogenesis is best described as
- **A.** the sequence of events by which spermatogonia are transformed into primary spermatocytes
- **B.** the sequence of events in which spermatocytes are derived from Sertoli cells
- **C.** the maturation of spermatocytes to spermatids
- **D.** the sequence of developmental events by which spermatids are transformed into mature sperm
- **E.** the first stage of spermatogenesis

**102.** The release of pepsinogen is the function of which of the following cells?
- **A.** parietal cells
- **B.** mucus cells
- **C.** Paneth cells
- **D.** enteroendocrine cells
- **E.** chief cells

**103.** That portion of the nephron unit whose cells have the most extensive brush border is the
- **A.** ascending limb of the loop of Henle
- **B.** distal convoluted tubule
- **C.** collecting tubule
- **D.** proximal convoluted tubule
- **E.** arched collecting tubule

**104.** Each of the following is an important characteristic of epithelia **EXCEPT**
- **A.** protection
- **B.** vascularity
- **C.** absorption
- **D.** secretion
- **E.** cell junctions

**105.** Growth in the diameter of a long bone is due to
   **A.** interstitial expansion of cartilage within the epiphyseal plate
   **B.** bone synthesis by the endosteum
   **C.** bone deposition by the periosteum
   **D.** secondary ossification centers
   **E.** appositional growth of the cartilage of the epiphyseal plate

**106.** The most generalized type of connective tissue (in the sense of possessing the greatest variety of connective tissue components) is
   **A.** adipose
   **B.** reticular
   **C.** loose
   **D.** mesenchymal
   **E.** dense irregular

**107.** Each of the following is required by the cell in the synthesis and packaging of proteins for export (secretion) **EXCEPT**
   **A.** Golgi apparatus
   **B.** smooth endoplasmic retiulum
   **C.** rough endoplasmic reticulum
   **D.** ribosomes
   **E.** nucleolus

**108.** Which of the following is associated directly with euchromatin?
   **A.** site of translation
   **B.** stains strongly basophilic
   **C.** smooth endoplasmic reticulum
   **D.** transcription
   **E.** stains strongly acidophilic

**109.** A cartilage surface not covered by a perichondrium
   **A.** is characteristic of elastic cartilage
   **B.** cannot exhibit interstitial growth
   **C.** is articular cartilage
   **D.** grows by apposition
   **E.** is never seen in adult humans

**110.** A lymphatic organ that filters blood is the
   **A.** spleen
   **B.** tonsil
   **C.** lymph node
   **D.** Peyer's patches
   **E.** thymus

**111.** Purkinje fibers
   **A.** are found in smooth and cardiac muscle
   **B.** serve functionally as connective tissue
   **C.** conduct impulses from smooth to skeletal muscle
   **D.** are part of an impulse-conducting system in the heart
   **E.** lack myofibrillae

**112.** The node of Ranvier is a region that may best be described as
   **A.** an area of sensory input
   **B.** a region where two Schwann cells are in juxtaposition
   **C.** a motor endplate
   **D.** an area covered with thick layers of smooth muscle
   **E.** an area for synaptic contact

**113.** The central component of the unit membrane consists primarily of
   **A.** potassium
   **B.** phospholipid
   **C.** calcium
   **D.** smooth endoplasmic reticulum
   **E.** proteins

**114.** Which of the following makes the ground substance of loose connective tissue homogeneous?
   **A.** hyaluronic acid
   **B.** collagen
   **C.** reticulum fibers
   **D.** elastic fibers
   **E.** laminin

**115.** The primary component of basal laminae is
   **A.** reticular fibers
   **B.** fibrils

  **C.** type I collagen
  **D.** type IV collagen
  **E.** tropocollagen

**116.** The major impediment to regeneration in the central nervous system is
  **A.** astrocytic processes
  **B.** oligodendroglial processes
  **C.** fibroblastic processes
  **D.** axonal processes
  **E.** collagen scar

**117.** The highest concentration of microtubules in neurons occurs at the
  **A.** endoplasmic reticulum clusters (of Nissl)
  **B.** apical dendrite
  **C.** initial segment of the axon
  **D.** node of Ranvier
  **E.** myelin sheath

**118.** The pacinian corpuscle
  **A.** is not responsive to mechanical stimulation
  **B.** is found only in joints and ligaments
  **C.** does not possess a lamellar structure of concentrically layered cells and fibers
  **D.** does not contain a sensory nerve ending
  **E.** is not responsive to vibrations

**119.** The iris is an internal part of the eye that
  **A.** is located posterior to the crystalline lens
  **B.** contains a muscle called the sphincter pupillae which dilates the pupil
  **C.** contains no pigment epithelium
  **D.** consists of a single layer of stratified squamous epithelium
  **E.** reduces the amount of light entering the eye and increases the depth of field when constricted by the sphincter pupillae

**120.** The aqueous humor
  **A.** is contained only within the anterior chamber of the eye
  **B.** serves only to provide support for the cornea
  **C.** is produced by a trabecular meshwork called the spaces of Fontana
  **D.** is drained by the canal of Schlemm
  **E.** is not important in maintaining normal intraocular pressure

**121.** Lymphatic nodules are found in each of the following **EXCEPT**
  **A.** lymph nodes
  **B.** the thymus
  **C.** the tonsils
  **D.** the spleen
  **E.** the walls of the urinary tract

**122.** Each of the following parts of the ear is surrounded by perilymph **EXCEPT**
  **A.** the utricle
  **B.** the cochlear duct
  **C.** the malleus
  **D.** the saccule
  **E.** the endolymphatic duct

**123.** A part of the uterine endometrium that remains relatively unchanged during the menstrual cycle is the
  **A.** stratum basalis
  **B.** stratum spongiosa
  **C.** stratum compacta
  **D.** surface epithelium
  **E.** endometrial blood vessels

**124.** Transitional epithelium prevents urine from leaking out of the bladder because of its
  **A.** gap junctions
  **B.** tight junctions
  **C.** desmosomes
  **D.** termal web
  **E.** glycocalyx

**125.** The primary source of ovarian progesterone is the
  **A.** corpus luteum
  **B.** stromal cells
  **C.** Graffian follicle
  **D.** corpus albicans
  **E.** cumulus oophorus

**126.** The two most abundant types of leukocytes in peripheral blood are
  **A.** lymphoctyes and monocytes
  **B.** neutrophils and lymphocytes
  **C.** neutrophils and basophils
  **D.** eosinophils and neutrophils
  **E.** lymphocytes and eosinophils

**127.** Collateral sprouting occurs in
  **A.** damaged axons
  **B.** damaged muscular tissue at the neuromuscular junctions
  **C.** intact glial processes
  **D.** damaged cell bodies
  **E.** undamaged axons

**128.** During erection of the penis, the volume of the blood occupying the spaces of the cavernous sinuses is increased by
  **A.** contraction of the musculature of the dorsal artery of the penis
  **B.** relaxation of the musculature of the dorsal artery of the penis
  **C.** relaxation of the musculature of the helicine arteries
  **D.** contraction of the musculature of the helicine arteries
  **E.** dilation of the smaller peripheral cavernous sinuses

**129.** Specializations of the surfaces of epithelial cells that permit the passage of low-molecular-weight particles through the cell membranes of contiguous cells are
  **A.** gap junctions
  **B.** tight junctions
  **C.** desmosomes
  **D.** not known to exist in mamalian tissues
  **E.** junctional complexes

**130.** Regarding the contents of their secretory vesicles, basophils of circulating blood are most similar to which of the following connective-tissue cell types?
A. histiocytes
B. fibroblasts
C. plasma cells
D. mast cells
E. reticular cells

**131.** A transverse section through the I-band of a sarcomere of skeletal muscle would include
A. actin myofilaments only
B. myosin myofilaments only
C. both actin and myosin myofilaments
D. Z-lines and actin myofilaments
E. H-bands, actin, and myosin myofilaments

**132.** The smallest molecules in the blood not filtered by the kidney are probably held back by the
A. capillary endothelium
B. slit membrane of the podocytes
C. basal lamina of the capillary
D. basal lamina of the podocytes
E. parietal layer of Bowman's capsule

**133.** Relative to the structure of the liver lobule, which of the following is correct?
A. it is arranged as a polygonal prism
B. the central vein runs at the periphery of the lobule
C. the portal vein runs through the center of the lobule
D. in humans there are well-developed connective-tissue partitions
E. branches of the hepatic artery are at the periphery of the lobule

**134.** The ability of skeletal muscle fibers to regenerate following injury is best described as
A. nonexistent
B. quite limited
C. moderately well developed

    **D.** extensive

    **E.** comparable to that of most epithelia

**135.** In traveling from the tympanic membrane to the hair cells of the organ of Corti, vibrations are conducted through each of the following **EXCEPT**

    **A.** the vestibular membrane

    **B.** perilymph

    **C.** endolymph

    **D.** the crista ampullaris

    **E.** the basilar membrane

**136.** Each of the following are features of the small intestine **EXCEPT**

    **A.** paneth cells

    **B.** villi

    **C.** goblet cells

    **D.** plicae circulares

    **E.** parietal cells

**137.** Oxygenated blood to the hepatic lobule is carried by the

    **A.** portal vein

    **B.** hepatic artery

    **C.** bile duct

    **D.** central vein

    **E.** hepatic vein

**138.** The hypothalamo-hypophyseal tract

    **A.** runs primarily from the hypothalamus to the pars nervosa

    **B.** is a double set of capillaries (sinusoids) separated by vessels of larger caliber

    **C.** carries no hormones

    **D.** carries releasing factors to the pars anterior

    **E.** begins in the pars anterior

**139.** Each of the following events occurs between the time of ovulation and menstruation **EXCEPT**

    **A.** high levels of progesterone appear in the secretory phase

    **B.** the uterine glands secrete glycogen

    **C.** the coiled arteries constrict

    **D.** high levels of estrogen appear in the ischemic phase

    **E.** the uterine glands become corkscrewlike in appearance

**140.** Each of the following parts of the nephron are lined with simple squamous epithelium **EXCEPT**
   A. the collecting tubule
   B. the proximal convoluted tubule
   C. Bowman's capsule
   D. the distal convoluted tubule
   E. the thin loop of Henle

**141.** Osteocytes of spongy bone are
   A. located within the organic bone matrix
   B. associated with Haversian systems
   C. derived from lymphocytes
   D. nourished via canaliculi
   E. responsible for bone absorption

**142.** The thyroid follicle is characterized by each of the following **EXCEPT**
   A. it is the structural unit of the thyroid gland
   B. it stores colloid
   C. it is made up of cuboidal follicular cells
   D. there is a major capillary bed
   E. it contains chief cells

**143.** The inner surface of the stomach is characterized by
   A. rugae
   B. villi
   C. crypts of Lieberkuhn
   D. plicae circulares
   E. Brunner's glands

**144.** Hyperparathyroidism, such as is produced by certain tumors of one or more of the parathyroid glands, would be expected
   A. to decrease blood calcium levels
   B. not to affect calcium metabolism
   C. to stimulate greater activity on the part of osteoclasts
   D. to increase the activity of osteoblasts
   E. to increase blood calcitonin levels

**145.** Lymphocytes are correctly described by each of the following **EXCEPT**
 A. they lack specific cyloplasmic granules
 B. they have a bilobed nucleus
 C. they may give rise to plasma cells
 D. they are divided into small and large cells
 E. they are responsible for immunologic memory

**146.** The endosteum of bone
 A. is traversed by Sharpey's fibers
 B. lines the medullary (marrow) cavity of long bones
 C. gives rise to the bony collar
 D. contains osteoclasts
 E. lines its external surface

**147.** A junctional complex typically includes
 A. a zonula occludens, a desmosome, and a zonula adherens
 B. a gap junction, a hemidesmosome, and a tight junction
 C. a tight junction, a basal lamina, and a terminal web
 D. a basal lamina, a hemidesmosome, and a gap junction
 E. a zonula occludens, a macula adherens, and a terminal web

**148.** After leaving the trabecular sinuses of a lymph node, lymph passes directly into the
 A. afferent lymphatic vessels
 B. efferent lymphatic vessels
 C. subcapsular sinuses
 D. medullary sinuses
 E. medulla

**149.** The main functional event at the neuromuscular junction is the
 A. interaction of calcium with troponin
 B. release of myosin from the prejunctional axolemma
 C. transmission of an electrical impulses to the Z line
 D. release of acetylcholine
 E. production of adenosine triphosphate (ATP)

**150.** Cartilage is found in each part of the respiratory tree **EXCEPT** the
  A. trachea
  B. primary bronchi
  C. respiratory bronchioles
  D. secondary bronchi
  E. tertiary bronchi

**151.** The function of the cell that has a basophilic cytoplasm, an eccentric nucleus, and a juxtanuclear Golgi apparatus is
  A. the synthesis of antibodies
  B. the release of histamine
  C. phagocytosis
  D. protein synthesis
  E. the synthesis of endorphins

**152.** A substance that is important in normal cell adhesion and migration is
  A. hyaluronidase
  B. procollagen
  C. fibronectin
  D. heparan sulfate
  E. phospholipid

**153.** The chemical in the granules of mast cells that results in vasodilation is
  A. heparin
  B. histamine
  C. phospholipid
  D. antibodies
  E. antigens

**154.** Which of the following layers in the wall of a medium-sized artery contains smooth muscle?
  A. the internal elastic membrane
  B. the tunica adventitia
  C. the external elastic membrane
  D. the tunica media
  E. the tunica intima

**155.** The most obvious histologic feature of the duodenum is the presence of
 A. serous cells
 B. Brunner's glands
 C. chief cells
 D. crypts of Lieberkühn
 E. Peyer's patches

**156.** At the pole of the renal corpusule, the juxtaglomerular cells are in direct contact with the
 A. proximal tubule
 B. loop of Henle
 C. efferent arteriole
 D. afferent arteriole
 E. distal tubule

**157.** The distal convoluted tubule of the kidney differs histologically from the proximal tubule by
 A. being more convoluted
 B. having taller columnar cells
 C. lacking a brush border
 D. having a smaller lumen
 E. having fewer cells in its wall

**158.** In compact bone, which of the following innerconnect the Haversian systems?
 A. Volkmann's canals
 B. interstitial lamellae
 C. concentric lamellae
 D. lacunae
 E. circumferential lamellae

**159.** The function of the parafollicular cells of the thyroid gland is to secrete
 A. thyroxin
 B. thyroglobulin
 C. parathormone
 D. calcitonin
 E. triodothyronine

**160.** The presence of Peyer's patches is characteristic of the
- **A.** esophagus
- **B.** jejunum
- **C.** duodenum
- **D.** cecum
- **E.** ileum

**161.** Which of the following layers of the meninges of the brain contains the blood vessels?
- **A.** arachnoid
- **B.** endosteal dura mater
- **C.** pia mater
- **D.** dura mater
- **E.** meningeal dura mater

**162.** The presence of microvilli on a cell usually indicates that the cell fuctions in
- **A.** neurotransmission
- **B.** collagen formation
- **C.** absorption
- **D.** hormone production
- **E.** secretory activities

**163.** Hassal's corpuscles are diagnostic for histologic sections of the
- **A.** tonsil
- **B.** saliva
- **C.** spleen
- **D.** thymus
- **E.** parathyroid

**164.** The tongue can be most readily identified by
- **A.** mucous glands
- **B.** stratified squamous epithelium
- **C.** mixed mucous and serous glands
- **D.** skeletal muscle disposed in three different planes
- **E.** mixed smooth and skeletal muscle

**165.** Which of the following segments of the nephron is essential for producing a hypertonic urine?
- **A.** the proximal convoluted tubule
- **B.** the thin segment of the loop of Henle

    **C.** the distal convoluted tubule
    **D.** Bowman's capsule
    **E.** the thick segment of the loop of Henle

**166.** Acid phosphatase can be used as a chemcal marker for the identification of centrifugal fractions of
    **A.** mitochondria
    **B.** nuclei
    **C.** microsomes
    **D.** lysosomes
    **E.** nucleoli

**167.** Adhering to the outer surface of the limiting membrane of the granular endoplasmic reticulum is/are the
    **A.** mitochondria
    **B.** lysosomes
    **C.** ribosomes
    **D.** Golgi complex
    **E.** centrioles

**168.** Which of the following makes up the striated, or brush, border?
    **A.** tightly packed cilia
    **B.** microtubules
    **C.** microvilli
    **D.** tonofibrils
    **E.** stereocilia

**169.** Myoepithelial cells are associated with the
    **A.** parotid gland
    **B.** submandibular gland
    **C.** pancreas
    **D.** sweat gland
    **E.** glands of von Ebner

**170.** Respiratory exchange of $O_2$ and $CO_2$ takes place in the
    **A.** primary bronchus
    **B.** terminal bronchiole
    **C.** trachea
    **D.** alveolar sacs
    **E.** lobar bronchus

**171.** The usual arrangement in most organs of an inner circular and outer longitudinal layer of smooth muscle is reversed in the wall of the
   A. stomach
   B. jejunum
   C. ureter
   D. gallbladder
   E. ileum

**172.** Multinucleate cells are frequently associated with the
   A. distal convoluted tubule
   B. parotid duct
   C. liver
   D. gallbladder
   E. esophagus

**173.** Podocytes are associated with which of the following parts of the urinary system?
   A. distal convoluted tubule
   B. urinary bladder
   C. major calyces
   D. thick limb of the loop of Henle
   E. visceral layer of Bowman's capsule

**174.** About 80% of the sodium and water filtered from the blood in the renal corpuscle is resorbed by the
   A. thin limb of the loop of Henle
   B. distal convoluted tubule
   C. thick limb of the loop of Henle
   D. proximal convoluted tubule
   E. collecting tubule

**175.** Filiform papillae are indicative of the
   A. epiglottis
   B. skin
   C. tongue
   D. stomach
   E. ileum

**176.** The basophils of the pars distalis of the pituitary gland secrete
A. thyrotropic hormone
B. oxytocin
C. growth hormone
D. prolactin
E. follicle-stimulating hormone

**177.** Each of the following is found within the cytoplasm of the nerve cell body **EXCEPT**
A. lysosomes
B. microtubules
C. ribosomes
D. Nissl's substance
E. axolemma

**178.** Each of the following distinguishes a section of the small intestine from that of the large intestine **EXCEPT**
A. villi
B. more goblet cells
C. glands of Brunner
D. Peyer's patches
E. plicae circulares

**179.** The spleen
A. acts as a filtering organ for blood
B. produces erythroctyes in the adult
C. produces lymphocytes
D. acts as a filtering organ for lymph
E. produces hormones

**180.** The proximal convoluted tubule is actively involved in the resorption of each of the following **EXCEPT**
A. glucose
B. water
C. sodium
D. amino acids
E. high-molecular-weight proteins

**181.** Which of the following characterizes the prostate gland?
- **A.** it serves as a storage gland for sperm
- **B.** it is formed by six to eight simple tubular glands
- **C.** it lacks a definite connective-tissue capsule
- **D.** it is the main source of acid phosphatase in the semen
- **E.** it is not affected by hormone levels

**182.** Which one of the following sensory receptors is responsible for proprioception?
- **A.** muscle spindles
- **B.** Ruffini's endings
- **C.** free nerve endings
- **D.** Meissner's corpuscles
- **E.** pacinian corpuscles

**183.** Cells that secrete lysozyme, which has antibacterial activity, are
- **A.** goblet cells
- **B.** chief cells
- **C.** parietal cells
- **D.** Paneth cells
- **E.** membranous epithelial cells

**184.** The following cells are commonly found in the thymus and are important in mediating immune reactions
- **A.** B lymphocytes
- **B.** plasma cells
- **C.** T lymphocytes
- **D.** monocytes
- **E.** erythrocytes

---

**DIRECTIONS (Questions 185–188):** The group of questions below consists of five lettered headings followed by a list of numbered words or statements. For each numbered word or statement, select the **one** lettered heading that is most closely associated with it. Each lettered heading may be selected once, more than once, or not at all.

---

    **A.** Pancreas
    **B.** Thymus
    **C.** Suprarenal gland
    **D.** Palatine tonsil
    **E.** Thyroid gland

**185.** Has crypts of stratified squamous epithelium covering lymph nodules

**186.** Has an exocrine portion that is under the influence of gastrointestinal hormones

**187.** Undergoes "age involution"

**188.** Has medullary cells that are derived from the neuroectoderm

---

**DIRECTIONS (Questions 189–218):** Each group of questions below consists of a list of numbered structures associated with figures. For each numbered structure, select the lettered item that identifies the structure in the figures.

---

**Questions 189–194:** Identify the lettered structures in the schematic representation of renal corpuscle (see Figure 9).

**189.** Parietal layer of Bowman's capsule

**190.** Proximal convoluted tubule

**191.** Glomerular capillary

**192.** Visceral layer of Bowman's capsule and podocytes

**193.** Afferent arteriole

**194.** Urinary space

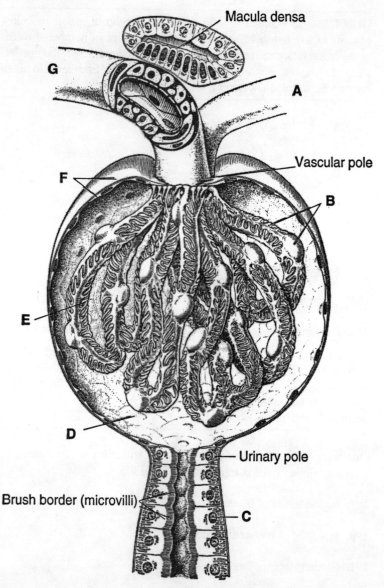

**Figure 9** Renal corpuscle. (Modified from Junqueira LC, et al.: *Basic Histology*, 7th ed. Norwalk, CT: Appleton & Lange, Inc, 1992.)

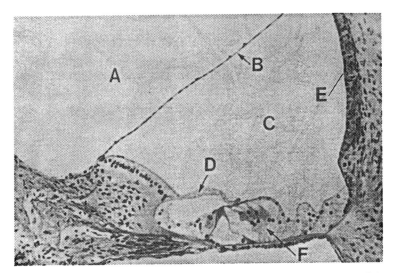

**Figure 10** Micrograph of the cochlea. (From Wilson JE. *Anatomy*, 9th ed. New York: Elsevier, 1991, p. 134).

**Questions 195–199:** Identify the lettered structures in the micrograph of the cochlea (see Figure 10).

**195.** Vestibular membrane

**196.** Stria vascularis

**197.** Tectorial membrane

**198.** Cochlear duct

**199.** Hair cells

**Questions 200–203:** Identify the lettered structures in the micrograph of the larynx (see Figure 11).

**200.** Vocalis muscle

**201.** Vocal (true) folds

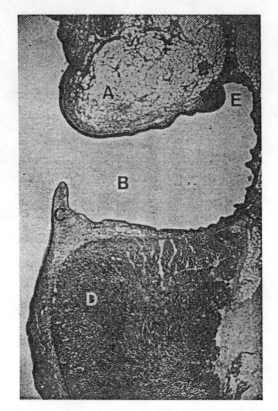

**Figure 11** Micrograph of the larynx. (From Wilson JE. *Anatomy,* 9th ed. New York: Elsevier, 1991, p. 136.)

**202.** Ventricle

**203.** Ventricular (false) folds

**Questions 204–208:** Identify the lettered structures in the schematic representation of a cell (see Figure 12).

**204.** Chromatin

**205.** Plasma membrane

**206.** Golgi apparatus

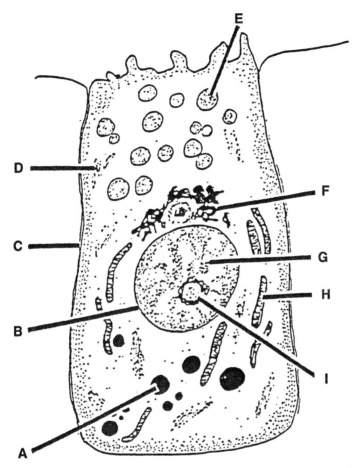

**Figure 12** Schematic picture of a cell. (From Wilson JE. *Anatomy,* 9th ed. New York: Elsevier, 1991, p. 137.)

**207.** Secretory granules

**208.** Nucleolus

**Questions 209–213:** Identify the structures at the epiphyseal plate (see Figure 13).

**209.** Hypertrophic cartilage zone

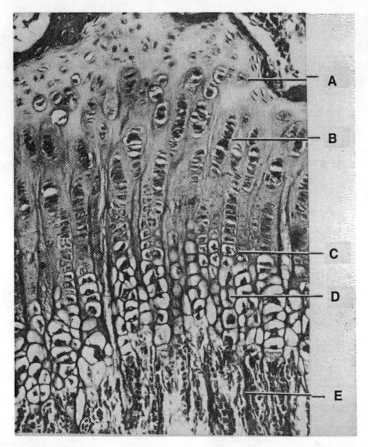

**Figure 13** Micrograph of the epiphyseal plate. (Modified from Junqueira LC, et al.: *Basic Histology*, 7th ed. Norwalk, CT: Appleton & Lange, Norwalk, 1992.)

**210.** Resting zone

**211.** Calcified cartilage zone

**212.** Proliferative zone

**213.** Ossification zone

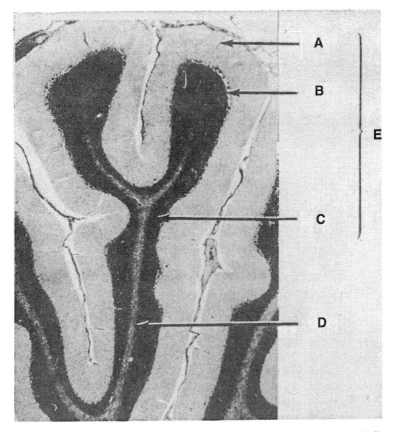

**Figure 14** Micrograph of the cerebellum. (Modified from Junqueira LC, et al.: *Basic Histology,* 7th ed. Norwalk, CT: Appleton & Lange, 1992.)

**Questions 214–218:** Identify the structures of the cerebellum (see Figure 14).

**214.** Gray matter

**215.** Granular layer

**216.** Molecular layer

**217.** Purkinje cell layer

# Microanatomy

## Answers and Comments

1. **(D)** The oligodendrocyte in the central nervous system is homologous to the Schwann cell in the peripheral nervous system. Both types of cells are found in gray and white matter, and function in myelination in the central nervous system. (**Ref. 3,** p. 172)

2. **(C)** During the proliferative phase of the menstrual cycle, there is a two- to threefold increase in the thickness of the endometrium. This phase is also called the follicular stage because ovarian follicles develop that produce estrogen, which stimulates cellular proliferation. (**Ref. 3,** p. 452)

3. **(E)** The polysaccharide products of the cell are synthesized by the Golgi apparatus, which consists of cisternae, vesicles, and vacuoles, and is usually located on the plasma membrane side of the nucleus. (**Ref. 3,** pp. 38–39)

4. **(B)** Tropocollagen, the structural unit of collagen, is synthesized by fibroblasts. Collagen is the most abundant protein of the body, with five major types described. Tropocollagen is the protein that polymerizes to from collagen. (**Ref. 3,** pp. 98–100)

5. **(B)** The interstitial cells (Leydig cells) of the testis secrete the hormone testosterone. These cells develop at puberty in the inter-

stitial tissue. Testosterone is responsible for the development of the secondary sex characteristics. (**Ref. 3**, p. 433)

6. **(E)** The heavy meromyosin of the muscle bundle is most closely associated with adenosine triphosphatase (ATPase) activity. The heavy meromyosin is the globular part of the rodlike molecules. (**Ref. 3**, p. 201)

7. **(D)** The mitochondria are the organelles that supply energy for the numerous reactions within cells. They accumulate at the part of the cell in which there is increased metabolic activity, and are composed mostly of protein. (**Ref. 3**, pp. 31–32)

8. **(B)** The cell organelle that plays an important role in the intracellular digestion of phagocytosed particles is the lysosome. It contains a number of hydrolytic enzymes that digest cytoplasmic macromolecules. The enzymes are produced in the rough endoplasmic reticulum. (**Ref. 3**, pp. 39–40).

9. **(A)** The Golgi apparatus has been shown to be a site for the concentration of secretory products. Condensing vacuoles develop and bud from the Golgi cisternae, forming vesicles for transportation. (**Ref. 3**, pp. 38–39)

10. **(E)** The respiratory bronchiole differs from the terminal bronchiole in having a few pulmonary alveoli in its wall. It also has cuboidal epithelium between the alveoli. Cilia are present in the proximal portion but not distally. Smooth muscle fibers and elastic fibers are well developed. Cartilage and glands are lacking. (**Ref. 3**, p. 346)

11. **(C)** Microglia are small cells distributed in the gray and white matter. These cells can change into phagocytic macrophages and remove necrotic tissue following damage to the central nervous system. (**Ref. 3**, p. 172)

12. **(C)** Intramembranous ossification begins in the second month of gestation in areas of loose mesenchyme. Capillaries grow into the mesenchyme, where the cells differentiate into osteoblasts. (**Ref. 3**, p. 150)

**13. (A)** Myelin is formed by Schwann cells rotating around the axon until numerous layers of the Schwann cell membrane surround the axon. The axon myelin is composed of a lipoprotein complex. (**Ref. 3,** p. 174)

**14. (C)** The granules in the cells of the adrenal medulla, which are innervated by preganglionic sympathetic neurons, contain epinephrine and norepinephrine. The cortex secretes glucocorticoids, mineralcorticoids, and androgens. (**Ref. 3,** pp. 407–409)

**15. (D)** The tunica vasculosa of the eye consists of the choroid, ciliary body, and iris. The sclera forms part of the outer or supporting layer of the eye and is composed of dense connective tissue. (**Ref. 3,** p. 471)

**16. (E)** Synapses may be classified on the basis of membrane specialization, organelle content, position, and variations in the quality and quantity of the synaptic vesicles of the axon terminal. The shape of the end bulb is not indicative of a type of synapse. (**Ref. 3,** pp. 169–170)

**17. (D)** The Merkel endings are classified as nonencapsulated nerve endings and are found in the deep layer of the epidermis. Each of the other receptors are highly or lightly encapsulated. (**Ref. 3,** pp. 357–363)

**18. (A)** In the secretory stage of the menstrual cycle there is hypertrophy of the endometrium. This enlargement is due mainly to increased vascularity and hypertrophy of the gland cells. (**Ref. 3,** p. 452)

**19. (C)** Adenosine triphosphate (ATP) is the critical energy source required by the muscle cell to contract. Each of the other changes is apparent during the contraction of skeletal muscle fibers. (**Ref. 3,** pp. 202–203)

**20. (C)** Most of the female urethra is lined by stratified squamous epithelium containing mucous glands. The lamina propria is thick and has abundant elastic tissue and veins. Smooth muscle fibers are found in the muscular layer. (**Ref. 3,** p. 392)

**21. (B)** The ductus deferens has a highly developed muscular coat consisting of three layers, and which contracts for the expulsion of sperm. The longitudinal folds in the lamina propria and epithelium result in a lumen with an irregular outline in cross section. The epithelium is pseudostratified columnar epithelium with stereocilia. (**Ref. 3**, p. 436)

**22. (D)** The rod cells are the taller cells in the retina and are very important in night vision. Rod cells contain the pigment rhodopsin, which responds to low intensities of light. In the center of the macula lutea is a region called the fovea centralis, which contains only closely packed cones. The cone cells are important in color vision. (**Ref. 3**, p. 481)

**23. (A)** Two types of nucleic acids are present in cells: ribonucleic acid (RNA) and deoxyribonucleic acid (DNA). Both are polymers of nucleotides, which are in turn composed of purine or pyrimidine and a phosphate group. DNA is found only in the nucleus, while RNA is present in both the nucleus and cytoplasm. (**Ref. 3**, pp. 54–55)

**24. (C)** The endoplasmic reticulum, as seen under the electron microscope, consists of a continuous network of membrane-bound cavities within the cytoplasm of nearly all cells. Two types of endoplasmic reticulum are recognized: the rough or granular type has ribonucleoprotein or ribosomes adhering to the outer surface of its limiting membrane, while the granular or smooth type lacks ribosomes. (**Ref. 3**, pp. 34–38)

**25. (C)** During metaphase, the mitotic spindle becomes larger and the centrioles are clearly visible at the poles. The chromosomes line the equatorial plane of the spindle. Toward the latter part of metaphase, the chromosomes undergo a longitudinal splitting, forming two identical chromatids. (**Ref. 3**, p. 59)

**26. (E)** In the adult, each organ has a characteristic type of epithelium which, under normal conditions, does not change. Under certain conditions, such as chronic inflammation or in the formation of tumors, one type of epithelium may change into another. This type of change is defined as metaplasia. (**Ref. 3**, p. 80)

**27. (E)** The cells of simple cuboidal epithelium, on a surface view, look like six-sided polygons, and on a vertical view look like a single even row of square cells whose height and thickness are about equal. This type of epithelium is found in many glands, on the free surface of the ovary, the inner surface of the capsule of the lens, the excretory ducts of numerous glands, and in the pigmented epithelium of the retina. (**Ref. 3,** p. 65)

**28. (D)** Simple columnar ciliated epithelium is limited in its distribution. It is usually found where the movement of luminal contents is necessary, as in the oviduct or smaller bronchi. It also occurs in the uterus, some of the paranasal sinuses, and lining the central canal of the spinal cord. (**Ref. 3,** p. 173)

**29. (E)** The red blood cells or erythrocytes of mammals are highly differentiated, nonmotile cells. They have lost their nuclei, Golgi apparatus, mitochondria, RNA, and centrioles during maturation. Their color is pale greenish-yellow in the living state. Hemoglobin is the oxygen-carrying pigment that gives erythrocytes their red color. (**Ref. 3,** pp. 234–237)

**30. (B)** Neuroglia or glial cells are found within the central nervous system. Histologically, one can distinguish four types of neuroglia: astroctytes, oligogdendrocytes, microglia, and ependymal cells. Microglia are of mesodermal origin, while the other types are ectodermal. (**Ref. 3,** pp. 170–174)

**31. (C)** In the large elastic arteries in humans, the basement membrane is very prominent. The endothelium consists of a single layer of polygonal cells and the tunica media is largely elastic tissue, consisting of 50 to 65 concentric elastic membranes. Relatively speaking, the tunica adventitia is thin. Bundles of smooth muscle cells are found in both the tunica intima and the media. (**Ref. 3,** p. 224)

**32. (E)** Sinusoids differ from capillaries in having a wide, irregular lumen and a very tenuous connective-tissue layer between the vascular wall and the organ. Sinusoids are usually lined with phagocytic cells, and thus belong to the reticuloendothelial system. These vascular channels are limited in their distribution to the spleen, liver, bone marrow, adrenal gland, and pituitary. (**Ref. 3**, p. 221)

33. (**E**) The thymus is a lymphatic organ that produces T-lymphocytes and consists of a cortex and medulla. The difference between the two parts is in the proportion of their lymphocyte as compared to reticular cell content. The cortex has many packed lymphocytes and a few reticular cells. The medulla has an opposite composition. The medulla is also more vascular and contains the characteristic thymic corpuscles or Hassall's bodies. Efferent lymphatics leave the thymus. (**Ref. 3**, pp. 265–268)

34. (**E**) The parotid gland is the largest of the salivary glands and is entirely serous. It is classified as a compound tubuloalveolar gland and has many ducts. The cells contain numerous secretory granules. The gland is enclosed in a thick, connective-tissue capsule. (**Ref. 3**, p. 312)

35. (**B**) The contraction of skeletal muscle depends on the presence of calcium. Following depolarization, the cisternae of the sacroplasmic reticulum release calcium close to the thick and thin filaments. (**Ref. 3**, p. 202)

36. (**E**) Nissl bodies are basophilic granular areas formed by rough endoplasmic reticulum. The bodies are arranged in parallel cisternae and are abundant in large nerve cells. (**Ref. 3**, p. 166)

37. (**C**) Neutrophils form about 60 to 70% of circulating leukocytes. They have a multilobed nucleus. Neutrophils have a short lifespan and are active in phagocytosis of bacteria throughout the body. (**Ref. 3**, pp. 237–239)

38. (**A**) The esophageal mucosa consists of stratified squamous epithelium beneath which is a lamina propria of loose connective tissue. A distinct muscularis mucosa is present. The glands of the esophagus are found in two sites: the esophageal glands proper are located in the submucosa and the cardiac glands in the lamina propria. The esophagus is enclosed in a layer of loose connective tissue called the tunica adventitia. (**Ref. 3**, p. 289)

**39. (B)** The size of the lumen of the bronchiole is controlled by elastic fibers and smooth muscle, which are found in the lamina propria. The smooth muscle is under control of the autonomic nervous system. (**Ref. 3,** p. 346)

**40. (C)** Three types of cells can be identified on the basis of their staining reaction in the pars distalis. These are acidophils, basophils, and chromophobes. These cells secrete hormones that regulate most endocrine glands, the secretion of milk, and muscle and bone metabolism. (**Ref. 3,** p. 399)

**41. (C)** The parathyroid glands secrete a polypeptide hormone, parathormone, which plays an important role in regulating the calcium concentration of the blood. The chief cells of the parathyroid gland secrete parathorome. (**Ref. 3,** pp. 420–422)

**42. (B)** Melanoblasts migrate from their origin in the neural crest to the stratum germinativum of the epidermis. Melancytes differentiate from melanoblasts. The subsequent differentiation of melanocytes into melanosomes is accompanied by the production of tyrosinase, which is necessary for the production of melanin. The melanin pigment in melanocytes can be identified through its staining reaction with the dopa reagent. (**Ref. 3,** p. 362)

**43. (D)** The subcapsular (marginal) sinus of a lymph node contains reticular fibers and cells, macrophages, and lymphocytes. Erythrocytes are not normally found in lymph nodes. (**Ref. 3,** pp. 269–272)

**44. (D)** The interstitial cells of Leydig are located in the stroma between the seminiferous tubules produce testosterone. These cells have an extensive smooth endoplasmic reticulum. Proteinaceous crystals (of Reinke) are also found. The production of testosterone is under the control of pituitary luteinizing hormone (LH). (**Ref.** p. 433)

**45. (D)** Semen is composed of seminal plasma, spermatozoa, and cast-off cells from the lining of the reproductive tract. The seminal plasma consist of secretions from the prostate, bulbourethral glands, seminal vesicles, and epididymis. The spermatozoa are produced by the seminiferous tubules. (**Ref. 3,** p. 423)

**46. (A)** The bile produced by the hepatic cells of the liver is first secreted into the bile canaliculi. The canaliculi coalesce as they leave the corresponding lobes of the liver to eventually form the right and left hepatic ducts. The two hepatic ducts unite to form the common hepatic duct, which joins the cystic duct to form the common bile duct. The common bile duct empties into the second part of the duodenum. (**Ref. 3,** p. 333)

**47. (C)** The glands of Von Ebner are associated with the trenches of the circumvallate papillae of the tongue. These glands drain into the goove at the base of each papilla and are important in keeping the taste bulbs clear. (**Ref. 3,** p. 284)

**48. (D)** The fibers of the periosteum that are embedded in the outer layer of compact bone are known as Sharpey's fibers. These fibers firmly anchor the periosteum to bone. (**Ref. 3,** p. 144)

**49. (D)** Surfactant produced by type II alveolar cells reduces surface tension, thus allowing expansion of the pulmonary alveoli. Premature infants may fail to produce sufficient surfactant and exhibit the respiratory distress syndrome. These infants do not have normally developed type II alveolar cells. (**Ref. 3,** pp. 349–350)

**50. (B)** The contraction or elastic recoil of the elastic tissue in the walls of the pulmonary alveoli is responsible for expelling air from the lungs. Patients with emphysema have impairment of this elastic tissue and consequent difficulty in expelling the alveolar contents. (**Ref. 3,** pp. 348–350)

**51. (B)** The cortical labyrinth of the kidney contains the renal corpuscles, proximal convoluted tubules, distal convoluted tubules, and arched collecting tubules. (**Ref. 3,** p. 371)

**52. (E)** The esophagus is unique in containing both skeletal and smooth muscle. The skeletal muscle is involuntary and is innervated by the vagus nerve. The first third of the esophagus contains mainly skeletal muscle, the middle third a mixture of both types of muscle, and the distal third primarily smooth muscle. (**Ref. 3,** p. 289)

53. **(A)** Based on the closed theory of circulation in the spleen, blood in the penicillar arteries enters into the sinusoids. These sinusoids drain into trabecular veins to reach the venous circulation. The open theory states that the penicillar arteries drain into the reticular meshwork between the sinusoids. (**Ref. 3,** pp. 273–276)

54. **(E)** Spongy bone has large, trabeculated soft tissue spaces whose volume exceeds the volume of the bone matrix. Compact bone has a larger volume of bone matrix than soft tissue spaces. (**Ref. 3,** p. 146)

55. **(B)** The pancreas is described as consisting of acinis (centroacinar cells) with central nuclei. These cells drain into an intercalated duct system that opens into intralobular ducts and ultimately into the pancreatic duct. (**Ref. 3,** pp. 317–320)

56. **(A)** Chief cells produce the digestive enzymes of the gastric secretions (pepsin and lipase). They are most concentrated in the bases of the fundic, gastric, and zymogenic glands. (**Ref. 3,** p. 296)

57. **(D)** Hydrochloric acid is produced by the parietal cells of the zymogenic glands of the stomach. The parietal cells also secrete an intrinsic factor required for the absorption of vitamin $B_{12}$. (**Ref. 3,** p. 294)

58. **(C)** All of the statements describing the male reproductive system are correct except that mature sperm are transferred through the vas deferens by peristaltic contractions of its muscular coat rather than by the movement of cilia. (**Ref. 3,** p. 436)

59. **(E)** The motility of mature sperm is based on the active movement of the flagellum and tail. The ATP necessary for this movement is produced in the mitochondrial sheath. (**Ref. 3,** pp. 424–428)

60. **(B)** Identification of muscle cells is based on the cell shape and the number and position of the cell nuclei. Skeletal muscle cells are cylindrical with tapered ends, and contain many peripheral nuclei. Cardiac muscle fibers are not tapered but appear to branch.

Their nuclei occupy a central position. Smooth muscle cells have a single, central nucleus and are long and tapered. (**Ref. 3,** p. 195)

61. (**A**) The neuromuscular junction is characterized by the presence of sarcolemmal folds (junctional folds) that invaginate into the sarcoplasm. They contain extensions of the synaptic clefts. (**Ref. 3,** pp. 203–206)

62. (**C**) The flat cells of the stratum granulosum in thick skin are characterized by the presence of keratohyalin granules. These granules stain deeply with hematoxylin and are stellate in shape. (**Ref. 3,** p. 358)

63. (**A**) Sebaceous and sweat glands are similar only in that both are part of the epidermis. Their functions and secretions are not the same. In addition, sweat glands are simple tubular glands while sebaceous glands are holocrine glands. (**Ref. 3,** pp. 357–363)

64. (**D**) The vascular pole of the renal corpuscle has afferent and efferent arterioles. The afferent vessel is derived from the intralobular arteries and supplies the glomerulus. The efferent arteriole drains the glomerulus into the capillary beds that surround the distal convoluted tubules. (**Ref. 3,** p. 371)

65. (**B**) The urinary bladder is lined with transitional epithelium that accommodates the stretching of the bladder during its filling with urine. (**Ref. 3,** p. 391)

66. (**D**) The vagina and esophagus are similar in that both are lined by stratified squamous epithelium, as is typical of epithelial surfaces that require protection. There are no glands in the vagina. Both the vagina and esophagus have various muscular layers in their walls. (**Ref. 3,** pp. 289, 459)

67. (**A**) The uterine tubes, uterus, and cervix have a simple columnar epithelial lining, while the vagina has a lining of stratified squamous epithelium. (**Ref. 3,** pp. 448–451)

68. (**C**) During follicular development, the ovarian follicle contributes progressively to the formation of the zona pellucida and the granulosa and thecal cells. After ovulation, the corpus luteum

is formed. Luteinizing hormone is produced by the pituitary gland. (**Ref. 3,** pp. 461)

69. **(B)** If fertilization does not occur, the corpus luteum involutes and is replaced by a scar tissue called the corpus albicans. This structure produces no hormones. (**Ref. 3,** p. 448)

70. **(C)** The growth of hyaline cartilage involves both interstitial and appositional growth. These processes provide a model for endochondral but not intramembranous bone formation. The primary growth of cartilage is appositional, depending on the development of chondrocytes from the cells of the perichondrium. (**Ref. 3,** pp. 137–138)

71. **(D)** The portal triads are located at the periphery of the liver lobules and contain a branch of the hepatic portal vein, proper hepatic artery, bile duct, and lymphatics. The central vein is located at the center of the lobule. (**Ref. 3,** p. 320)

72. **(A)** The kidney is divided into an outer cortex and an inner medulla. The cortex contains the glomeruli and the proximal and distal convoluted tubules. The loop of Henle is located in the medulla (**Ref. 3,** pp. 371–373)

73. **(B)** The two proteins actin and myosin are responsible for the contractile activity of muscle cells. Actin exists in the form of a thin filament and myosin as a thick filament. (**Ref. 3,** pp. 47–49)

74. **(E)** Recent evidence suggests that the transport of sperm through the female reproductive tract results from the peristalsis of the uterus and oviduct rather than the movement of cilia or fluid movement. (**Ref. 3,** p. 453)

75. **(C)** Neutrophils are active in the acute inflammatory response. Following injury, neutrophils migrate from the vascular system and engulf bacteria by phagocytosis. This process also engulfs particles from the surrounding tissue. (**Ref. 3,** pp. 109–110)

76. **(B)** Drug detoxification occurs primarily in the liver, with the smooth endoplasmic reticulum being the part of the cell that functions in the breakdown of drugs. (**Ref. 3,** pp. 36–38)

**77. (C)** The rough endoplasmic reticulum is the membranous organelle that secretes proteins. Ribosomes are bound to the rough endoplasmic reticulum. **(Ref. 3, p. 35)**

**78. (A)** Mitochondria are referred to as the "powerhouse" of the cell because this is where the cellular oxidation process occurs. A chain of enzymes are necessary for the conversion of adenosine monophosphate (AMP) to ATP. **(Ref. 3, pp. 31–33)**

**79. (D)** Lysosomes are membranous organelles that contain hydrolytic enzymes (acid hydrolases). These organelles are functionally important in defense and autolysis of the cell and in breaking down ingested proteins by phagocytosis. Protein production is a function of the rough endoplasmic reticulum. **(Ref. 3, pp. 39–43)**

**80. (E)** Stratified squamous keratinizing epithelium is the typical epithelium in skin, where the outer layer of keratin serves to waterproof the skin and protect it from wear and injury. This type of epithelium also protects the body by blocking the penetration of bacteria through the skin. **(Ref. 3, p. 76)**

**81. (D)** Leukocytes are divided into two major categories based on the staining reaction of their cytoplasmic granules. There are three types of granular leukocytes (eosinophils, basophils, and neutrophils) and two types of nongranular leukocytes (lymphocytes and monocytes). **(Ref. 3, p. 237)**

**82. (B)** Platelets are small cytoplasmic fragments that lack a nuclear component. Following an injury, platelets from the circulating blood adhere to the inner surface of the vessel wall, resulting in platelet aggregation and blood coagulation. The platelet count is increased by thrombopoietin. **(Ref. 3, pp. 245–247)**

**83. (A)** In a longitudinal section, skeletal muscle fibers show a pattern of dark (A band) and light (I band) striations. Z-lines bisect the I bands. The sarcomere comprises each of these three components of muscle fibers. **(Ref. 3, pp. 197–200)**

84. **(E)** The sarcoplasmic reticulum is an organelle in the muscle fiber that is responsible for regulating the concentration of calcium ions within the myofibrils. (**Ref. 3,** p. 202)

85. **(C)** Cardiac muscle is the only type of muscle that has a spontaneous, inherent ability to contract without any autonomic nerve supply. Cardiac muscle has central nuclei, striations, and intercalated discs. (**Ref. 3,** pp. 208–211)

86. **(B)** Smooth muscle fibers are characterized by three contractile filaments, but do not have the same sarcomere arrangement as skeletal or cardiac muscle. Smooth and cardiac muscle cells are innervated by the autonomic nervous system. (**Ref. 3,** pp. 211–214)

87. **(C)** Plasma cells are most commonly found in connective tissue and lymphatic tissue. They have an eccentric nucleus and contain an abundance of ribosomes. Plasma cells are active in protein secretion and the production of humoral antibodies. (**Ref. 3,** pp. 113–116)

88. **(B)** Macrophages (histiocytes) are typical cells of connective tissue. They are rich in lysosomes and very active in the phagocytosis of foreign matter. They are an essential part of the reticuloendothelial system and do not produce collagen. (**Ref. 3,** pp. 108–111)

89. **(A)** Connective tissue contains three types of fibers: collagen, elastic, and reticular. Collagen fibers are thick and unbranched and are made up of fibrils. Elastic fibers are thin and branched and appear slightly yellow. Reticular fibers are not very prominent and are made up of fine and delicate branched fibers. (**Ref. 3,** p. 120)

90. **(E)** The precursor of collagen is a protein called procollagen, which is produced by the rough endoplasmic reticulum. The alpha chains of procollagen are similar to collagen molecules and can be synthesized in 5 or 6 minutes. (**Ref. 3,** p. 101)

91. **(A)** Cartilage is an avascular tissue; the nutrition of chondrocytes within its lacunae occurs by the diffusion of nutrient materi-

als through the matrix from capillaries outside the cartilage. (**Ref. 3**, p. 132)

92. **(A)** Cartilage is a gel-like ground substance that contains collagen fibrils made of type II collagen, which add strength to the cartilage. In addition, about one-half of the cartilage matrix consists of cartilage proteoglycan produced by chondrocytes. (**Ref. 3**, p. 134)

93. **(D)** The oppositional growth of cartilage involves the deposition of more cartilage on the existing cartilage surface by cells in the chondrogenic layer of the perichondrium, which lay down new cartilage matrix. (**Ref. 3**, pp. 137–138)

94. **(C)** The inorganic components of bone make up 75% of its dry weight, with calcium phosphate and calcium carbonate constituting about 95% of this weight. (**Ref. 3**, pp. 143–144)

95. **(C)** The Haversian system (osteons) are formed by concentric lamellae of bone that have a Haversian canal at their center. The canals are lined with osteogenic cells and run parallel with the long axis of the bone. (**Ref. 3**, p. 148)

96. **(B)** The thymus develops from the third and fourth branchial pouches of the pharynx. In this development, reticular cells derived from epithelial cells arrange themselves in a loose network of cells connected by desmosomes. (**Ref. 3**, p. 266)

97. **(B)** The paracortical region of the lymph node and periarterial sheaths of the spleen are considered to be thymus-dependent regions because each undergoes rapid depletion of T- and B-cells following neonatal thymectomy. (**Ref. 3**, pp. 269, 273)

98. **(D)** The adventitia is the thickest layer of a large vein. This layer contains bundles of collagen and elastic fibers, and often contains longitudinal bundles of smooth muscle fibers (**Ref. 3**, p. 226)

99 **(A)** Fenestrated capillaries have thin, attenuated regions with permanent fenestrae between the endothelial cells. The fenestrae

are covered by a very thin diaphragm and are irregularly spaced. (**Ref. 3,** p. 220)

100. **(B)**   The two most commonly found cells in the islet of Langerhans are the beta and alpha cells. The beta cells are the most numerous and produce a polypeptide hormone, insulin. Glucagon is produce by the alpha cells. (**Ref. 3,** pp. 410–413)

101. **(D)**   Spermiogenesis is the last phase of spermatogenesis, in which the rounded spermatids transform into spermatozoa. During this process, changes occur in the Golgi region and nucleus. (**Ref. 3,** p. 424)

102. **(E)**   The granules of the chief cells of the stomach contain the enzyme pepsinogen. With the release of this enzyme into the acidic stomach, pepsinogen is converted to pepsin. (**Ref. 3,** p. 296)

103. **(D)**   The luminal border of the proximal convoluted tubules is covered with dense microvilli that form what is called the brush border. This border provides the increased surface area necessary for the active resorptive function of the proximal tubules. The other components of the duct system do not have any significant number of microvilli on their luminal borders. (**Ref. 3,** pp. 378–381)

104. **(B)**   Epithelia are described by each of the listed characteristics except for vascularity. Epithelia contain no capillaries, but receive their nourishment by diffusion from the adjacent loose connective tissue. (**Ref. 3,** pp. 66–73)

105. **(C)**   Increase in the diameter of a long bone is due to the growth of osteoblasts from the cells of the periosteum. These cells form lamellae of bone on the outer surface of the bone. The growth in length occurs at the epiphyseal plate. (**Ref. 3,** pp. 154–156)

106. **(C)**   Loose connective tissue is found in almost every aspect of the body surrounding nerves, vessels, muscles, and viscera. It is much more general in location than the other types of connective tissue listed. (**Ref. 3,** p. 120)

**107. (B)** The smooth endoplasmic reticulum is devoid of ribosomes and is prominent in only a few cell types. Smooth endoplasmic reticulum does not synthesize protein, but is involved in the synthesis of lipids and detoxification of drugs. (**Ref. 3,** pp. 36–38)

**108. (D)** Euchromatin is the extended, active form of chromatin that provides the instructions for such cellular functions as protein secretion. Gene transcription occurs from extended chromatin, for which euchromatin is necessary. (**Ref. 3,** p. 54)

**109. (C)** Articular cartilage is a smooth surface of cartilage that lacks a perichondrium. Therefore, all growth is interstitial and not by apposition. Articular cartilage is sustained by nutrients diffused from the synovial fluid. (**Ref. 3,** p. 132)

**110. (A)** The spleen is the only structure listed that filters blood by phagocytic removal of lipid droplets and old and damaged cells. The spleen also has other functions, including the degradation of hemoglobin and production of lymphocytes. (**Ref. 3,** pp. 228–278)

**111. (D)** Purkinje fibers are specialized muscle fibers that conduct the impulses for myocardial contraction more rapidly than does ordinary heart muscle. Purkinje fibers are found primarily in the deepest area of the myocardium. (**Ref. 3,** pp. 228–229)

**112. (B)** Nodes of Ranvier represent interruptions of the myelin sheath that surrounds myelinated nerve fibers along their length. These nodes are found on nerves in the central and peripheral nervous system. It is at these nodes that the nerve fiber undergoes depolarization. (**Ref. 3,** p. 177)

**113. (B)** The unit membrane or plasma membrane is a three-layered structure of which the middle layer comprises phopholipids. The plasma membrane functions as a selective barrier and regulates passage of materials in and out of the cell. (**Ref. 3,** pp. 26–27)

**114. (A)** The homogeneous nature of ground substance is due to glycoproteins and a number of glycosaminoglycans, such as hyaluronic acid. (**Ref. 3,** pp. 94–95)

**115. (D)** Type IV collagen is the primary collagen in basal laminae. This type of collagen consists of a glycoprotein known as laminin and proteoglycan. (**Ref. 3,** p. 68)

**116. (A)** Following damage to the central nervous system, astrocytes proliferate and cause scar tissue that impedes the regeneration of nerve tissue. This replaces the connective tissue that develops after damage to other tissues of the body. (**Ref. 3,** pp. 185–188)

**117. (C)** The initial segment of an axon emerges from the cell body at the axon hillock, where the cell contains many microtubules and neurofilaments with little rough endoplasmic reticulum. (**Ref. 3,** p. 168)

**118. (E)** Pacinian corpuscles are encapsulated receptors that are widely distributed throughout the dermis and in joint capsules. They are oval in shape and surrounded by concentric lamellae of cells. The pacinian corpuscles are responsive to mechanical stimulation and also can detect vibrations. (**Ref. 3,** pp. 467–468)

**119. (E)** The iris is the diaphragm located between the anterior and posterior chambers of the eye. The iris is covered by two to three layers of pigmented cells. Pupillary size is regulated by the sphincter and dilator pupillae muscles, which decrease and increase the size of the pupil, respectively. (**Ref. 3,** p. 470)

**120. (D)** The aqueous humor is the watery fluid formed in the ciliary processes and which fills the anterior and posterior chambers of the eye, as well as providing nutrients to the cornea and lens. The balanced volume of this fluid maintains normal intraocular pressure. From the anterior chamber the fluid drains into the canal of Schlemm to reach the venous blood. (**Ref. 3,** pp. 471, 476)

**121. (B)** Lymphatic nodules are aggregates of small lymphocytes found in the intestines, respiratory tract, urinary tract, lymph nodes, tonsils, and spleen. The thymus contains no lymphatic nodules in its cortex or medulla. (**Ref. 3,** pp. 269–279)

**122. (C)** The malleus is in the middle ear cavity, which is filled with air. The other structures are found in the bony labyrinth of the inner ear, where there is a fluid-filled environment of perilymph. (**Ref. 3,** p. 490)

123. **(A)** The basal layer of the uterus is not affected during the menstrual cycle because it has its own separate blood supply, unlike the other parts of the uterus. (**Ref. 3,** p. 452)

124. **(B)** Tight junctions allow transitional epithelium to withstand stretching without the cells pulling apart. This makes this type of epithelium well adapted for lining viscera that are subject to distention. (**Ref. 3,** p. 391)

125. **(A)** The corpus luteum develops after rupture of the ovarian follicle. A blood clot forms initially, after which the granulosa lutein cells are formed. It is these cells that make most of the progesterone produced by the corpus luteum. (**Ref. 3,** p. 448)

126. **(B)** The most abundant leukocyte found in peripheral blood is the neutrophil (50 to 70%). These cells are important in the acute inflammatory reaction. The second most numerous cell is the lymphocyte (20 to 50%), which is functionally important for the immune system. (**Ref. 3,** pp. 237–241)

127. **(E)** Collateral sprouting is characteristic of normal, healthy axons. The branches formed by this process usually leave the axon almost perpendicularly and then make a right-angled turn. (**Ref. 3,** p. 169)

128. **(C)** Erection is a parasympathetic response that results primarily from the relaxation off the smooth muscle in the walls of the arteries (helicine arteries) that supply the cavernous bodies of the penis. (**Ref. 3,** p. 439)

129. **(A)** Gap junctions are membrane separations that create narrow intercellular gaps of about 3 nm. These gaps allow the passage of ions and small molecules directly from one cell to another. (**Ref. 3,** pp. 71–73)

130. **(D)** Basophils and mast cells are similar in that both release an inflammatory mediator into the bloodstream following an antigenic stimulus. If the mediator is released in large quantities,

it can cause widespread vascular collapse and death. (**Ref. 3,** p. 241)

131. (**A**)   The I bands consist only of thin filaments that contain actin. The Z line bisects the I band, and myosin myofilaments are found in the thick filaments of the A band. (**Ref. 3,** pp. 197–201)

132. (**B**)   The endothelial pores of the glomerular capillaries filter cellular elements from the blood. The basal lamina of the visceral layers of Bowman's capsule filters macromolecules, while the smallest molecules, that are prevented from entering the intracapsular space, are probably held back by the slit membranes of the podoctyes. (**Ref. 3,** pp. 387–390)

133. (**A**)   The liver is the largest gland in the body. Its structural and functional unit is the liver lobule. In histologic sections, the lobules of the liver are arranged as polygonal prisms or hexagons. Within the center of each lobule runs the central vein, while at the periphery can be found branches of the portal vein, hepatic artery, and bile duct. This triad is called a portal canal. Connective-tissue partitions separating the lobules are not well developed. The radially arranged liver cells are situated on each side of the liver sinusoids. (**Ref. 3,** pp. 320–321)

134. (**B**)   Skeletal muscle has a limited ability to regenerate following injury. Satellite cells are thought to be the only source of the new myoblasts that can form new muscle cells. Most damaged muscle fibers are replaced by fibrous scar. (**Ref. 3,** p. 214)

135. (**D**)   The cristae ampullaris are located in the semicircular ducts, and are involved in the transmission of impulses of rotational acceleration and deceleration of the head. The other structures are involved in the transmission of sound impulses. (**Ref. 3,** p. 490)

136. (**E**)   Parietal cells are located in the gastric pits of the stomach, and are responsible for the production of acid. Each of the other structures is characteristic of the small intestines. (**Ref. 3,** pp. 297–306)

137. (**B**)   The hepatic artery carries oxygenated blood to the hepatic lobule. The blood in the portal vein comes from the intestines and

spleen. The central vein drains blood from the lobule to the hepatic veins and inferior vena cava. (**Ref. 3,** p. 323)

**138. (A)** The hypothalamo-hypophyseal tract is an axon fiber tract that begins at the cell bodies in the hypothalamus and extends to the pars nervosa of the pituitary. Oxytocin and vasopressin are carried by this tract. (**Ref. 3,** pp. 394–397)

**139. (D)** Estrogen production is most prominent during the proliferative stage of the menstrual cycle, in which there is active regrowth of the endometrium. Little estrogen is present in the ischemic phase of the cycle. (**Ref. 3,** pp. 451–453)

**140. (A)** The collecting tubules are lined with cuboidal or columnar cells, while the other components of the nephron are lined with simple squamous epithelium. (**Ref. 3,** pp. 371–378)

**141. (D)** Osteocytes develop from osteoblasts within the bone lacunae connected by canaliculi. Diffusion of oxygen and nutrients to the osteocyte occurs through these channels. (**Ref. 3,** p. 142)

**142. (E)** Chief cells are found in the parathyroid glands and produce parathyroid hormone. Thyroid follicles contain cuboidal cells that are surrounded by an extensive capillary bed. The follicles store colloid or thyroglobulin. (**Ref. 3,** p. 414)

**143. (A)** Rugae are longitudinal folds of the mucosa of the stomach. Villi, crypts, plicae circulares, and Brunner's glands are features of the small intestine. (**Ref. 3,** pp. 289–293)

**144. (C)** The increased levels of parathyroid hormone resulting from a tumor increased the blood calcium concentration. This hormone primarily targets the osteoblasts that function in bone resorption. (**Ref. 3,** pp. 420–422)

**145. (B)** Lymphocytes have a spherical nucleus and lack cytoplasmic granules. These cells play an important role in the immune response. Bilobed nuclei are typical of eosinophils. (**Ref. 3,** pp. 241–245)

**146. (B)** The endosteum is a layer of osteogenic cells that lines the internal cavities of long bones. The osteogenic cells can proliferate into osteoblast or chondryoblasts. (**Ref. 3**, p. 144)

**147. (A)** A junctional complex consists of three kinds of junctions: the zonula occludens, zonula adherens, and desmosome. The three junctions are responsible for binding cells together. (**Ref. 3**, p. 73)

**148. (D)** Lymph enters the node via the afferent lymphatics that drain through the subcapsular sinus to the cortical sinuses before reaching the medullary sinuses. (**Ref. 3**, pp. 269–272)

**149. (D)** On the axon terminals of the neuromuscular junction are many synaptic vesicles that contain acetylcholine. Depolarization of these axon terminals causes the release of acetylcholine. (**Ref. 3**, p. 203)

**150. (C)** Cartilage is found in the respiratory tree from the trachea to the primary, secondary, and tertiary bronchi. Bronchioles are characterized by a lack of cartilage or glands. (**Ref. 3**, pp. 345–348)

**151. (A)** The plasma cell under the light microscope is seen to contain an eccentric, rounded nucleus and small nucleolus. Its heterochromatic material is arranged in a cartwheel manner next to the nuclear membrane. The cytoplasm is strongly basophilic. The major function of the plasma cell is the production and release of antibodies. (**Ref. 3**, pp. 113–116)

**152. (C)** Fibronectin is a high-molecular-weight glycoprotein produced by fibroblasts. It helps to maintain normal cell adhesion and migration. (**Ref. 3**, p. 96)

**153. (B)** Histamine is found in the granules of mast cells and assists in initiating the acute inflammatory reaction. It causes the smooth muscle of most arteries to relax and dilate, with the exception of the pulmonary and coronary arteries. (**Ref. 3**, pp. 111–113)

**154. (D)** The tunica media in the wall of medium-sized arteries contains smooth muscle. It can contain up to 40 layers of smooth muscle cells. It also contains some elastic and reticular fibers. (**Ref. 3,** p. 223)

155. **(B)**  Brunner's glands in the submucosa historically identify the duodenum. These glands secrete an alkaline, mucous product that protects the mucous membrane from acid juices. (**Ref. 3,** p. 303)

156. **(D)**  The juxtaglomerular cells are in contact on one side with the tunica intima of the afferent arteriole and on the other side with the base of the epithelial cells of the macula densa, which is found in the wall of the distal convoluted tubule. (**Ref. 3,** p. 385)

157. **(C)**  The distal convoluted tubule of the kidney differs histologically from the proximal convoluted tubule in that it lacks a brush border. The lumina of the distal tubules are also larger and more acidophilic. (**Ref. 3,** pp. 383–384)

158. **(A)**  Volkmann's canals interconnect the Haversian systems in compact bone. These canals run transversely and do not have concentric lamellae. The Volkmann's canals connect with the canals of the Haversian systems. (**Ref. 3,** p. 148)

159. **(D)**  Calcitonin is secreted by the perifollicular cells of the thyroid gland. These cells are part of the thyroid follicles and contain numerous small granules that store calcitonin, which is used to regulate calcium levels. (**Ref. 3,** p. 415)

160. **(B)**  Peyer's patches in the mucosa enable one to histologically identify the ileum. They consist of aggregates of lymphoid nodules in the submucosa. There are about 30 such patches in the ileum. (**Ref. 3,** p. 303)

161. **(C)**  The pia mater is the vascular meningeal layer of the brain and spinal cord. It is a loose connective-tissue layer lying directly on the surface of the brain and spinal cord. The pia mater forms tunnels traversed by blood vessels. (**Ref. 3,** p. 193)

162. **(C)**  Microvilli are characteristic of cells that are actively engaged in absorption. They project from the surface of the cell and are very numerous in aborptive cells because they increase the surface area of the mucosa. (**Ref. 3,** p. 74)

**163. (D)** Hassal's corpuscles consist of concentric arrays of squamous epithelial cells and are specific to the thymus. They are found in the medulla and degenerate and become filled with keratohyalin granules. (**Ref. 3,** p. 265)

**164. (D)** The unique arrangement of skeletal muscle in three different planes is characteristic of a section of the tongue. The planes of muscle are separated by connective tissue, with the mucosa tightly adherent to the muscle. (**Ref. 3,** p. 283)

**165. (B)** The thin segment of Henle's loop is essential for producing a hypertonic urine in the kidney, thus maintaining body water. Henle's loop concentrates urine as it flows through the ducts. (**Ref. 3,** p. 389)

**166. (D)** Acid phosphatase is used as a chemical marker in the identification of centrifugal fractions of lysosomes. These organelles contain acid phosphatase, which allows localization of this enzyme to such cells. (**Ref. 3,** p. 18)

**167. (C)** Ribosomes adhere to the outer surface of the limiting membrane of the granular endoplasmic reticulum. They are cytoplasmic organelles that function as the site of protein synthesis in the cell. (**Ref. 3,** pp. 33–34)

**168. (C)** Under the electron microscope, the striated or brush border seen under the light microscope is identified as microvilli. These are short or long fingerlike projections from the cell surface, and are more numerous on absorptive cells. (**Ref. 3,** p. 74)

**169. (D)** Myoepithelial cells are associated with sweat glands. They are located in the basal lamina and surround serous acini, where they are sometimes called basket cells. (**Ref. 3,** p. 312)

**170. (D)** Respiratory exchange of $O_2$ and $CO_2$ takes place in the alveolar sacs and alveoli. The alveolar wall is specialized for this function. The wall consists of two thin epithelial layers with capillaries and macrophages between these layers. (**Ref. 3,** p. 348)

**171. (C)** The layers of smooth muscle in the muscularis externa of the wall of the ureter consist of inner logitudinal and outer circular layers. These layers of the ureter blend with the muscle layers of the bladder. (**Ref. 3,** p. 392)

172. **(C)**   Multinucleate cells are occasionally seen among the cells of the liver. They are usually located close to the space of Disse, and contain one or two nuclei with one or two nucleoli. (**Ref. 3,** pp. 320–328)

173. **(E)**   The epithelial cells that constitute the visceral layer of Bowman's capsule are known as podocytes. The podocytes have processes called pedicels that encircle the glomerular capillaries. The pedicel of one podocyte will embrace several capallaries and touch the basal lamina. (**Ref. 3,** pp. 371–376)

174. **(D)**   Approximately 85% of the sodium and water filtered by the blood is resorbed by the proximal convoluted tubule of the kidney. This is the first site for absorption after the glomerulus and maintains fluid homeostasis for the body. (**Ref. 3,** p. 388)

175. **(C)**   The tongue is characterized by the presence of three types of papillae. These are the filiform, which are the most numerous, the fungiform, and the circumvallate. Taste buds are located on the latter two types of papillae. (**Ref. 3,** p. 283)

176. **(E)**   The basophils of the pars distalis of the pituitary gland secrete follicle stimulating hormone and luteinizing hormone. These cells are referred to as gonadotrophic cells. (**Ref. 3,** pp. 399–400)

177. **(E)**   The axolemma is the plasma membrane of the axon. All of the other components of the nerve cell are found in the cytoplasm of the cell body. (**Ref. 3,** p. 168)

178. **(B)**   The large intestine has more goblet cells. Each of the other features is characteristic of the small intestine. The villi and plicae circulares are found throughout both the large and small intestines. Brunner's glands are found only in the duodenum and Peyer's patches only in the ileum. (**Ref. 3,** pp. 306–308)

179. **(A)**   The spleen functions as a filtering organ for blood and plays a role in the iron metabolism of the body. It produces lymphocytes and is the largest lymphoid organ in the body. It is an im-

portant defense against microorganisms in the circulation. (**Ref. 3,** pp. 272–273)

**180. (E)** All of the glucose and 80% of the sodium and water in the glomerular filtrate are resorbed by the proximal convoluted tubule. Amino acids, ascorbic acid, and acetoacetic acid are also resorbed, as are low-molecular-weight proteins. (**Ref. 3,** pp. 388–389)

**181. (D)** The prostate gland consists of 30 to 50 small, compound tubulo-alveolar glands whose ducts open into the urethra. The secretion of the gland serves as a vehicle for the transport of sperm, and is the primary source of acid phosphatase and citric acid in the semen. The gland has a strong capsule and the gland changes size depending on hormone levels. (**Ref. 5,** pp. 437–438)

**182. (A)** The muscle spindles are encapsulated proprioceptors responsible for detecting the position of the body in space. These spindles have nerve fibers that penetrate the muscle, where they detect changes in the length of muscle fibers. (**Ref. 3,** p. 467)

**183. (D)** Paneth cells are located in the bases of the intestinal glands. They are exocrine serous cells that synthesize lysozyme, which can digest the cell walls of some bacteria. (**Ref. 3,** p. 301)

**184. (C)** T lymphocytes constitute 35% of circulating lymphocytes. They originate in the bone marrow and migrate to the thymus, where they produce large lymphoid cells called immunoblasts. These cells then differentiate into cells of the immune system. (**Ref. 3,** pp. 261–263)

**185. (D)** Specifically characteristic of the palatine and lingual tonsil are crypts lined by stratified squamous epithelium. Beneath the epithelium are numerous lymph nodules. The pharyngeal tonsil lacks crypts. (**Ref. 3,** pp. 279–280)

**186. (A)** The secretion of the exocrine portion of the pancreas is believed to be under the influence of gastrointestinal hormones called secretins. The exocrine portion of the pancreas is composed of serous cells that secrete several enzymes for digestion. (**Ref. 3,** pp. 317–320)

**187. (B)** The thymus is a lymphoid structure that reaches it maximum development before puberty. After puberty it involutes. It produces several protein growth factors that stimulate T-lymphocyte production. (**Ref. 3,** pp. 265–268)

**188. (C)** The medullary parenchymal cells of the adrenal medulla give rise to epinephrine and norepinephrine, and are derived from the neuroectoderm. They are innervated by preganglionic sympathetic fibers. (**Ref. 3,** p. 407)

**189. (F)** The parietal layer of the glomerular (Bowman's) capsule lines the outer wall of the renal corpuscle. It forms a simple squamous epithelial lining of the capsule, supported by a basal lamina and reticular fibers. (**Ref. 3,** p. 371)

**190. (C)** The proximal convoluted tubule is the largest part of the nephron and leaves the renal corpuscle at the tubular pole. It courses through the cortex and medulla and becomes the loop of Henle. (**Ref. 3,** pp. 378–379)

**191. (E)** The glomerular capillaries form loops that are attached to the vascular pole of the renal corpuscle and receive blood from the afferent arteriole. They are supported by a substantial basement membrane. (**Ref. 3,** p. 376)

**192. (B)** The visceral layer of the glomerular capsule is the epithelial covering of the glomerular capillary. It is continuous with the parietal layer of epithelium. Specialization of this layer forms podocytes and their processes. (**Ref. 3,** p. 371)

**193. (G)** The afferent arteriole is a branch of the intralobar arteries, which enter the renal corpuscle at the vascular pole. It supplies blood to the capillaries of the glomeruli. The blood leaves the glomeruli via the efferent arterioles. (**Ref. 3,** p. 386)

**194. (D)** The urinary space is the lumen of the renal corpuscle between the parietal and visceral layers. This space receives the fluid that filters through the capillary wall and visceral layer. (**Ref. 3,** p. 371)

**195. (B)** The vestibular membrane forms the roof of the cochlear duct, separating it from the scala vestibuli. The membrane is very thin, consisting of two layers of simple squamous epithelium. (**Ref. 3,** p. 492)

**196. (E)** The stria vascularis is a specialized vascularized epithelium that lines the cochlear duct and functions in the formation of endolymph. It consists of three cell types, with capillaries running between the cells. (**Ref. 3,** p. 492)

**197. (D)** The tectorial membrane is a sheet of protein that roofs over the hair cells. It is supported by the spiral lamina. The tips of the tallest outer hair cells are embedded in the membrane. (**Ref. 3,** p. 492)

**198. (C)** The cochlear duct (scala media) is an endolymph-filled membranous labyrinth of triangular shape. The basilar membrane forms the floor of the cochlear duct, supporting the organ of Corti and functioning as a sound receptor. (**Ref. 3,** p. 491–492)

**199. (F)** Hair cells are the specialized receptor cells in the organ of Corti, and are usually divided into outer and inner cell groups. Some of these cells have many efferent endings and others have cup-shaped endings at the base of the cell. (**Ref. 3,** p. 490)

**200. (D)** The vocalis muscle is the laryngeal muscle that lies just deep and lateral to the vocal ligament. This muscle parallels the vocal ligament and is responsible for fine pitch control. (**Ref. 3,** p. 345)

**201. (C)** The vocal fold is also known as the true focal fold and lies immediately inferior to the ventricle. The vocal fold is formed by the vocal ligament and the overlying stratified squamous epithelium. Vibration of these folds produces vocal sounds. (**Ref. 3,** p. 343)

**202. (B)** The ventricle is the chamber of the larynx between the vocal and ventricular folds. The most lateral extension of the ventricle is the saccule, in which mucus glands are located. (**Ref. 3,** p. 345)

**203.** (A) The ventricular or false vocal folds are found just superior to the ventricle. They are lateral and superior to the vocal folds and are more protective in function. (**Ref. 3,** p. 343)

**204.** (G) Chromatin is the basophilic material within the nucleus that forms the chromosomes and deoxyribonucleic acid (DNA). It exists in two forms: heterochromatin and euchromatin. (**Ref. 3,** pp. 54–57)

**205.** (C) The plasma membrane is the outer membrane covering of the cell. It has a trilaminar appearance, described as the unit membrane. It serves as a selective barrier and regulates the passage of some materials in and out of the cell. (**Ref. 3,** pp. 25–32)

**206.** (F) The Golgi apparatus is formed by layers of parallel sacs or vesicles. These are often located close to the nucleus and function in the accumulation and concentration of secretory products. (**Ref. 3,** pp. 38–39)

**207.** (E) Secretory granules or vesicles are bounded by a unit membrane that is used for the storage of secretory proteins. These are discharged when required. Most of these products are released by hormones or neural messages. (**Ref. 3,** p. 44)

**208.** (I) The nucleolus is a nuclear organelle that functions in the formation of ribosomal ribonucleic acid (RNA). It stains deeply basophilic. One to two nucleoli are observed in most cells. The nucleolus is divided into three parts: nucleolar-organizer DNA, the pars fibrosa, and the pars granulosa. (**Ref. 3,** p. 57)

**209.** (C) The hypertrophic cartilage zone is located in the midpart of the epiphyseal plate. It contains large chondrocytes with glycogen, and has thin septa between the chondrocytes. (**Ref. 3,** p. 153)

**210.** (A) The resting zone is the area closest to the epiphysis. It is composed of hyaline cartilage without any morphologic cellular differences. (**Ref. 3,** p. 153)

**211.** (D) The calcified cartilage zone develops with the death of chondrocytes. The thin septa of cartilage become calcified with the deposition of hydroxyapatite. (**Ref. 3,** p. 153)

212. **(B)** The proliferative zone is the area of most rapid bone growth. The chondrocytes in this zone divide rapidly. They exist in columns of cells that are parallel to the long axis of the bone (**Ref. 3,** p. 153)

213. **(E)** The ossification zone is the terminal part of the epiphyseal plate. Endochondral bone develops here, along with blood vessels and osteoblasts that deposit a calcified matrix. (**Ref. 3,** p. 153)

214. **(E)** The superficial layer of the cortex is the gray matter, which consists of three layers. These layers are the molecular layer, Purkinje cell layer, and granular layer. (**Ref. 3,** p. 190)

215. **(C)** The granular layer is the innermost layer of the cortex. The cells in this layer are very small, with three to six dendrites and a single axon. (**Ref. 3,** p. 191)

216. **(A)** The molecular layer is the most superficial layer of the cerebellum. It consists of unmyelinated nerve fibers and a few perikaryons. (**Ref. 3,** p. 191)

217. **(B)** The Purkinje cell layer is the intermediate layer of the cortex, between the molecular and granular layer. The Purkinje cells are very large, flask-shaped cells that have numerous dendrites that divide repeatedly. The axons of these cells form the beginning of the outflow of the cerebellum. (**Ref. 3,** p. 191)

218. **(D)** The white matter of the cerebellum is the central core of cerebellar nerve tissue. It contains nerve fibers and supporting neuroglial cells, but no cell bodies. (**Ref. 3,** pp. 189–191)

# 4

# Embryology

1. Closure of the foramen primum results from fusion of the
   A. septum secundum
   B. septum secundum and septum spurium
   C. septum primum and fused endocardial cushions
   D. septum secundum and fused endocardial cushions
   E. septum primum and sinoatrial valve

2. During the fourth week of development, the formation of the right and left atrioventricular canals results from the
   A. fusion of the dorsal and ventral endocardial cushions
   B. development of the interventricular septum
   C. fusion of the septum primum and septum secundum
   D. partitioning of the truncus arteriosus
   E. closure of the foramen ovale

3. The most common ventricular septal defect results from the
   A. transposition of the great vessels
   B. persistence of the truncus arteriosus
   C. failure of the aorticopulmonary septum to develop
   D. failure of development of the membranous part of the inter-
      ventricular septum
   E. absence of the muscular part of the interventricular septum

4. The ventral pancreatic bud develops into the
   A. neck of the pancreas
   B. common bile duct
   C. body of the pancreas
   D. uncinate process
   E. tail of the pancreas

5. Rotation of the intestinal loops of the midgut
   A. is 270° counterclockwise
   B. is 270° clockwise
   C. places the right vagus anterior to the stomach
   D. places the left vagus anterior to the stomach
   E. is around the axis of the inferior mesenteric artery

6. Which of the following is usually associated with an absence of
   the brain?
   A. macrocephalus
   B. hydrocephalus
   C. cranioschisis
   D. microcephalus
   E. conical cranium

7. Fusion of one or more fingers and toes is called
   A. syndactyly
   B. polydactyly
   C. meromelia
   D. amelia
   E. brachydactyly

8. The main pancreatic duct is derived
   A. partly from the dorsal pancreatic bud and partly from the
      ventral pancreatic bud
   B. entirely from the dorsal pancreatic bud

C. entirely from the ventral pancreatic bud
D. from neither of the pancreatic buds
E. entirely from the proximal part of the hepatic diverticulum

9. Meckel's diverticulum results from abnormal persistence of
   A. the allantois
   B. the yolk stalk
   C. herniated gut
   D. the urorectal system
   E. meconium

10. The site of the cloacal membrane (which is also the point of demarcation between endodermal and ectodermal epithelium) is represented in the adult by the
    A. rectal columns
    B. transition zone
    C. white line
    D. external anal sphincter
    E. anal valves (pectinate line)

11. Primordial germ cells arise in the
    A. coelomic epithelium overlying the genital ridge
    B. yolk sac mesoderm
    C. primary sex cords of the indifferent gonad
    D. yolk sac endoderm
    E. epiblastic layer of the embryonic disc

12. The ejaculatory ducts of the male develop from the
    A. caudal end of the mesonephric ducts
    B. cephalic end of the mesonephric ducts
    C. caudal end of the urogenital sinus
    D. cephalic end of the urogenital sinus
    E. allantois

13. The primary components of the male reproductive system develop from the
    A. paramesonephric ducts
    B. anorectal canal
    C. caudal end of the allantois
    D. metanephros
    E. mesonephric ducts

**14.** The paramesonephric duct in female embryos gives rise to the
  A. clitoris
  B. uterine tubes and uterus
  C. urethra
  D. round ligament of the uterus
  E. ovarian ligament

**15.** The medulla of the suprarenal gland derives from
  A. lumbar ectoderm
  B. gut endoderm
  C. mesoderm of the dorsal mesentery
  D. neural crest cells
  E. mesoderm of the ventral mesentery

**16.** Intervillous spaces are lined by
  A. uterine epithelium
  B. decidual cells
  C. cellular trophoblast
  D. syncytiotrophoblast
  E. chorionic mesoderm

**17.** The notochordal process is composed of
  A. embryonic ectoderm
  B. embryonic endoderm
  C. embryonic mesoderm
  D. extraembryonic ectoderm
  E. extraembryonic mesoderm

**18.** The myotomes that form most of the skeletal muscle mass of the body derive from
  A. lateral plate mesoderm
  B. splanchnic mesoderm
  C. ectoderm
  D. intermediate mesoderm
  E. paraxial mesoderm

**19.** The cloaca is divided into the rectum and urogenital complex by the
  A. cloacal membrane
  B. urogenital ridge

    **C.** sinal bulbs
    **D.** urorectal septum
    **E.** rectal columns

**20.** The anterior two-thirds of the tongue develop from the
    **A.** lateral lingual swellings
    **B.** second branchial arch
    **C.** tuberculum impar
    **D.** copula
    **E.** third branchial arch

**21.** The lower lip is formed from the
    **A.** maxillary prominences
    **B.** lateral nasal prominences
    **C.** mandibular prominences
    **D.** frontonasal prominence
    **E.** nasolacrimal groove

**22.** The major part of the definitive palate is formed by the
    **A.** intermaxillary segment
    **B.** lateral palatine processes
    **C.** frontal prominence
    **D.** primary palate
    **E.** second branchial arch

**23.** A cleft lip on the left side of the philtrum indicates failure of fusion of the
    **A.** left and right maxillary prominences
    **B.** left lateral nasal and left maxillary prominences
    **C.** left lateral and left medial nasal prominences
    **D.** medial nasal prominence and left maxillary prominence
    **E.** left medial nasal prominence and mandibular process

**24.** The principal activities of the placenta include each of the following **EXCEPT**
    **A.** exchange of gases
    **B.** exchange of nutrients
    **C.** transmission of maternal antibodies
    **D.** blood formation
    **E.** hormone production

**25.** Each of the following are features of monozygotic twins **EXCEPT**
   A. they result from the fertilization of one ovum
   B. they are of the same sex
   C. they are genetically identical
   D. two placentas
   E. usually two amnions

**26.** The first branchial arch gives rise to each of the following **EXCEPT** the
   A. anterior belly of the digastic muscle
   B. mylohyoid muscle
   C. malleus
   D. muscles of facial expression
   E. incus

**27.** The frontonasal prominence gives rise to the
   A. bridge of the nose
   B. cheeks
   C. lips
   D. mandible
   E. maxilla

**28.** The cloaca communicates with each of the following structures **EXCEPT** the
   A. mesonephric duct
   B. allantois
   C. amnion
   D. hindgut
   E. urogenital sinus

**29.** The mesoderm gives rise to each of the following **EXCEPT**
   A. cartilage
   B. bone
   C. the kidneys
   D. the suprarenal gland
   E. the urinary bladder

**30.** A cardiovascular malformation that involves the abnormal involution of the right fourth aortic arch and proximal right dorsal aorta between the right fourth aortic arch and seventh intersegmental artery is the
  **A.** right aortic arch
  **B.** retroesophageal right subclavian artery
  **C.** double aortic arch
  **D.** patent ductus arteriosus
  **E.** transposition of the great vessels

**31.** The valve of the foramen ovale is formed by the
  **A.** endocardial cushions
  **B.** lower part of the septum secundum
  **C.** upper end of the septum primum
  **D.** lower end of the septum primum
  **E.** ostium secundum

**32.** The aortic arch between the left common carotid and left subclavian artery is formed by the
  **A.** left fourth aortic arch
  **B.** right fourth aortic arch
  **C.** left sixth aortic arch
  **D.** right sixth aortic arch
  **E.** third aortic arch

**33.** The hepatic sinusoids develop from the
  **A.** anterior cardinal veins
  **B.** posterior cardinal veins
  **C.** supracardinal veins
  **D.** vitelline veins
  **E.** ductus venosus

**34.** At birth, the obliterated left umbilical vein forms the
  **A.** ligamentum venosum
  **B.** ligamentum teres hepatis
  **C.** ligamentum arteriosum
  **D.** inferior vena cava
  **E.** portal vein

**35.** A double superior vena cava results from the failure of the left brachiocephalic vein to form and the persistence of the

   **A.** subcardinal veins
   **B.** supracardinal veins
   **C.** common cardinal veins
   **D.** right posterior cardinal vein
   **E.** left anterior cardinal vein

**36.** Omphalocele can result from

   **A.** weakening or a defect in the musculature of the anterior abdominal wall
   **B.** failure of the gut loops to return to the abdomen
   **C.** secondary herniation of the gut
   **D.** defective formation of the diaphragmatic musculature
   **E.** failure of the right and left sternal halves to fuse

**37.** The gonadal sex of an individual is originally determined by the presence of

   **A.** androgens from the testis
   **B.** an anti-Müllerian hormone
   **C.** an ovary with follicles
   **D.** Sertoli cells
   **E.** a Y chromosome

**38.** The round ligament of the uterus is derived from the original

   **A.** broad ligament covering the uterus
   **B.** gubernaculum
   **C.** round ligament of the ovary
   **D.** suspensory ligament of the mesonephros
   **E.** urachus

**39.** The respiratory system develops as an outgrowth of the

   **A.** lateral lingual swellings
   **B.** tuberculum impar
   **C.** ventral wall of the foregut
   **D.** proximal end of the midgut
   **E.** first branchial arch

**40.** Respiratory distress syndrome occurs most commonly because
  A.  too few mature alveoli have developed
  B.  surfactant production is insufficient
  C.  the lungs are partially filled with amniotic fluid
  D.  type I alveolar epithelial cells produce a greatly thickened basement membrane
  E.  abnormally developed lung buds

**41.** Tetralogy of Fallot typically includes each of the following defects **EXCEPT**
  A.  an overriding aorta
  B.  a high ventricular septal defect
  C.  stenosis of the pulmonary trunk
  D.  right ventricular hypertophy
  E.  stenosis of the aortic semilunar valve

**42.** Which of the following is a vitellline duct anomaly?
  A.  umbilical hernia
  B.  omphalocele
  C.  umbilical fistula
  D.  gastroschisis
  E.  duodenal stenosis

**43.** The dorsal mensentery forms each of the following **EXCEPT** the
  A.  greater omentum
  B.  falciform ligament
  C.  dorsal mesoduodenum
  D.  transverse mesocolon
  E.  mesentery proper

**44.** Primordial germ cells are correctly described by each of the following **EXCEPT**
  A.  form primitive sex cords
  B.  first appear in the wall of the yolk sac
  C.  migrate along the dorsal mesentery of the hindgut
  D.  invade the genital ridges at the sixth week of development
  E.  induce development of a gonad into an ovary or a testis

45. Trisomy 21 is usually characterized by each of the following **EX-CEPT**
    A. mental retardation
    B. cleft palate
    C. congenital heart defects
    D. results from a nondisjunction of chromosomes
    E. simian creases in the hands

46. Bowman's capsule is formed by the
    A. metanephros
    B. ureteric bud
    C. pronephos
    D. metanephric mesoderm
    E. mesonephros

47. The bladder
    A. is a derivative of the hindgut
    B. is entirely derived from endoderm
    C. is formed entirely from mesoderm
    D. has dual origin from the urogenital sinus and mesonephric duct
    E. was not connected to the allantois during development

48. The origin of the urogenital system is most closely related developmentally to the
    A. paraxial mesoderm
    B. intermediate mesoderm
    C. lateral plate mesoderm
    D. splanchnic mesoderm
    E. somatic mesoderm

49. Derivatives of the ventral mesentery include each of the following **EXCEPT** the
    A. hepatoduodenal ligament
    B. falciform ligament
    C. mesocolon
    D. hepatogastric ligament
    E. visceral peritoneum of the liver

**50.** The inner layer of the invaginating optic vesicle differentiates into the
  A. lens placode
  B. neural retina
  C. cornea
  D. iris
  E. ciliary body

**51.** The sulcus limitans delineates the
  A. alar plate from the basal plate
  B. basal plate from the floor plate
  C. alar plate from the roof plate
  D. marginal layer from the mantle layer
  E. mantle layer from the ependymal layer

**52.** The first branchial pouch will develop into the
  A. external auditory meatus
  B. thymus gland
  C. middle ear cavity
  D. palatine tonsil
  E. inner ear

**53.** The origin of a high anorectal agenesis with a rectovesical fistula involves
  A. persistence of the anal membrane
  B. excessive resorption of the foregut
  C. defective urorectal septum
  D. hypoplasia of the infraumbilical mesoderm
  E. persistence of the allantois

**54.** The artery supplying most of the developing embryonic foregut is the
  A. celiac artery
  B. superior mesenteric artery
  C. inferior mesenteric artery
  D. umbilical artery
  E. internal thoracic artery

**DIRECTIONS (Questions 55–65):** Each group of questions below consists of five lettered headings followed by a list of numbered statements. For each numbered statement, select the **one** lettered heading that is most closely associated with it. Each lettered heading may be selected once, more than once, or not at all.

A. Intraembryonic mesoderm
B. Somatic mesoderm
C. Splanchnic mesoderm
D. Intraembryonic coelom
E. Pleuropericardial membrane

**55.** Forms the parietal layer of serous membranes

**56.** Forms the visceral layer of serous membranes

**57.** Forms the fibrous pericardium

**58.** Is continuous with the wall of the yolk sac

**59.** Forms cells that spread between the epiblast and hypoblast layers

A. Mesonephric duct
B. Ureteric bud
C. Metanephric mesoderm
D. Pronephros
E. Mesonephros

**60.** Gives rise to the ureter and renal pelvis

**61.** Gives rise to the loop of Henle

**62.** Together with the gonads forms the urogenital ridge

**63.** Gives rise to the glomeruli

**64.** Degeneration of this structure results in renal agenesis

**65.** Gives rise to the paroophroron in the female

# Embryology

## Answers and Comments

1. **(C)** The foramen primum develops between the septum primum and the fused endocardial cushions as the septum primum grows from the roof of the common atrium. Failure of these two structures to fuse would result in a patent foramen primum. (**Ref. 4,** p. 312)

2. **(A)** Initially there is a single atrioventricular canal. Dorsal and ventral endocardial cushions develop as swellings on the respective dorsal and ventral walls of the single atrioventricular canal. Growth of mesenchymal cells in these cushions results in their fusion and formation of the right and left canals. (**Ref. 4,** p. 312)

3. **(E)** The interventricular septum develops from a larger muscular part and a smaller, more superior membranous part. The most common ventricular septal defect is caused by failure of the membranous part to develop along with inadequate growth of the endocardial cushions. (**Ref. 4,** p. 330)

4. **(D)** The pancreas develops from the dorsal and ventral pancreatic buds that originate from the duodenum. The ventral bud forms the uncinate process and inferior head of the pancreas, with the remainder of the gland forming from the dorsal bud. (**Ref. 4,** pp. 244–245)

5. **(A)** Rotation of the midgut occurs partly during herniation into the umbilical cord (90°) and during return of the intestinal loops into the abdominal cavity (180°). The rotation is counterclockwise and occurs around the axis of the superior mesenteric artery. **(Ref. 4,** p. 248)

6. **(C)** Anomalies that involve the size and shape of the skull are identified by certain descriptive terms. Thus, acrania or cranioschisis, or open-roofed skull, is related to virtual absence of the brain. Microcephalus refers to a small cranium and undersized brain, while an abnormally large skull is a macrocephalus. **(Ref. 4,** p. 364)

7. **(A)** Several types of anomalies occur in the development of the extremities and digits. Failure of the limbs to develop is called amelia, while deficiency of a distal portion of a limb is called hemimelia. The presence of abnormally short digits is called brachydactyly. A union of adjacent digits is called a syndactyly, and polydactyly is indicated by a supernumerary digit. **(Ref. 4,** p. 378)

8. **(A)** The pancreas develops from ventral and dorsal pancreatic buds of endodermal cells that arise from the caudal part of the foregut that is developing into the proximal part of the duodenum. The main pancreatic duct forms from the duct of the ventral bud and the distal part of the duct from the dorsal bud. **(Ref. 4,** p. 244)

9. **(B)** Meckel's diverticulum of the ileum is one of the most common malformations of the digestive tract. This diverticulum represents the remnant of the proximal portion of the yolk stalk. The diverticulum can become inflamed and cause pain. **(Ref. 4,** p. 255)

10. **(E)** The inferior one-third of the anal canal develops from the proctodeum, while the superior two-thirds is derived from the hindgut. The junction of the epithelium derived from the endoderm of the hindgut and ectoderm of the proctodeum is indicated by the pectinate line at the level of the anal valves. **(Ref. 4,** p. 258)

11. **(D)** The primordial germ cells are seen early in the fourth week of development among the endodermal cells of the yolk sac, near

the origin of the allantois. During folding of the embryo, part of the yolk sac becomes incorporated into the embryo, and the primordial germ cells migrate to the gonadal ridges. (**Ref. 4,** p. 281)

12. **(A)** The caudal ends of the mesonephric ducts move medially to enter the prostatic urethra, where they become the ejaculatory ducts. The ducts develop between the seminal vesicle and the urethra. (**Ref. 4,** p. 288)

13. **(E)** The mesonephric ducts play a key role in development of the duct system of the testis, vas deferens, seminal vesical, and ejaculatory ducts. The mesonephric ducts come under the influence of testosterone in the eighth week of development. They degenerate almost completely in the female. (**Ref. 4,** p. 285)

14. **(B)** The paramesonephric ducts develop into the major genital duct system of the female and caudally form the uterine tubes and uterus. These ducts develops lateral to the mesonephric ducts. (**Ref. 4,** p. 285)

15. **(D)** Neural crest cells develop along the crest of each neural fold as the neural tube separates from the ectoderm. These cells migrate and give rise to a number of structures, including the suprarenal medulla. (**Ref. 4,** p. 63)

16. **(D)** Intervillous spaces develop from lacunar networks that are derived from syncytiotrophoblast during the second week. These spaces are filled with blood that enters them from the spiral arteries. (**Ref. 4,** p. 118)

17. **(C)** The embryonic mesodermal cells of the primitive streak and the primitive node form a cellular cord called the notochordal process. The process grows cranially between the ectoderm and endoderm until it reaches the prechordal plate. (**Ref. 4,** p. 57)

18. **(E)** The intraembryonic mesoderm on each side of the notochord divides into paraxial, intermediate, and lateral mesoderm. The paraxial mesoderm is adjacent to the neural tube and divides into paired somites in the third week of development. The somites split to form myotomes that further divide to form the skeletal muscles. (**Ref. 4,** pp. 63, 370)

244 / 4: Embryology

19. **(D)** The cloaca is divided by a wedge of mesenchyme called the urorectal septum. This septum grows caudally and forms folds that grow toward each other and fuse. The partition divides the cloaca into two parts: the rectum and upper anal canal dorsally and the urogenital sinus ventrally. (**Ref. 4,** p. 258)

20. **(A)** The two lateral lingual swellings develop on each side of and overgrow the tuberculum impar. They develop from the first pair of branchial arches and fuse to form the anterior two-thirds of the tongue. (**Ref. 4,** p. 203)

21. **(C)** The paired mandibular prominences form caudal to the stomodeum. During the fourth week of development they merge across the midline to form the lower lip and jaw. This is the first part of the face to form. (**Ref. 4,** p. 208)

22. **(B)** The secondary or definitive palate is formed by the midline fusion of the lateral palatine processes. The secondary palate is the primordium of the hard and soft palates posterior to the incisive foramen. (**Ref. 4,** p. 216)

23. **(D)** A left cleft lip is due to lack of fusion of the maxillary prominence with the fused medial nasal prominences. The clefts range from small notches to large defects. The lip is divided into medial and lateral parts. (**Ref. 4,** p. 221)

24. **(D)** Blood formation occurs early in the allantois and yolk sac and later in the liver. The principal activities of the placenta are endocrine secretion and the transfer of gases, nutrients, and antibodies. (**Ref. 4,** pp. 120–122)

25. **(D)** Monozygotic twins result from the feritlization of one ovum. As a result, these twins are of the same sex, are genetically identical, and are quite similar in appearance. They have two amniotic sacs and one placenta, whereas dizygotic twins have two placentas. (**Ref. 4,** p. 134)

26. **(D)** The first branchial arch gives rise to the muscles innervated by the mandibular division of the trigeminal nerve, to the malleus and incus, and to the sphenomandibular ligament. The muscles of

facial expression develop from the second branchial arch. (**Ref. 4,** p. 199)

27. **(A)** The frontonasal prominence gives rise to the bridge of the nose and to the forehead. This is a single process that surrounds the forebrain and gives rise to optic vesicles. The other structures develop from the maxillary and lateral nasal prominences. (**Ref. 4,** p. 208)

28. **(C)** The cloaca in the terminal part of the hindgut. It is separated from the surface ectoderm by the cloacal membrane. The cloaca communicates with the allantois, hindgut, urogenital sinus, and mesonephric duct. (**Ref. 4,** p. 258)

29. **(E)** The mesoderm gives rise to cartilage, bone, connective tissue, muscle, the heart, blood, lymph vessels and cells, the kidneys, gonads, genital ducts, serous membranes, the spleen, and the suprarenal glands. The urinary bladder develops from endoderm. (**Ref. 4,** pp. 74–75)

30. **(B)** The abnormal origin of the right subclavian artery is formed by the right seventh intersegmental artery and the persistence of the distal portion of the right dorsal aorta. The origin of the abnormal right subclavian artery is just below the left subclavian artery, and the artery crosses the midline behind the esophagus. (**Ref. 4,** p. 340)

31. **(D)** After the septum secundum has formed, the upper part of the septum primum regresses, with the lower part remaining as the valve of the foramen ovale. (**Ref. 4,** p. 312)

32. **(A)** The fate of the fourth aortic arch is different on the two sides of the body. On the right, the fourth arch forms the proximal right subclavian artery, and on the left it forms the aortic arch between the left common carotid and subclavian arteries. (**Ref. 4,** p. 335)

33. **(D)** The liver buds grow into the septum transversum and interrupt the plexus of vitelline veins to form a network of hepatic sinusoids. The hepatic cords anastomose to form the sinusoids. (**Ref. 4,** p. 243)

**34. (B)** At birth, the obliteration of the left umbilical veins forms the ligamentum teres hepatis in the falciform ligament. The closure of the ductus venosus forms the ligamentum venosum. **(Ref. 4, p. 341)**

**35. (E)** The persistent left anterior cardinal veins form the left superior vena cava, which drains into the coronary sinus. The right anterior and common cardinal veins form the normal superior vena cava on the right. **(Ref. 4, pp. 304–305)**

**36. (B)** An omphalocele is a persistence of the herniated abdominal contents into the proximal part of the umbilical cord. This occurs during the tenth week of development and usually involves only the intestines. **(Ref. 4, p. 251)**

**37. (E)** The embryo's chromosomal sex is determined by the type of sperm (X or Y) that fertilizes the ovum. An X sperm produces an XX zygote, which develops into a female, whereas a Y sperm produces an XY zygote, which develops into a male. **(Ref. 4, p. 32)**

**38. (B)** The gubernaculum is attached to the uterus. The cranial part of the gubernaclum becomes the ovarian ligament and the caudal part forms the round ligament, which passes through the inguinal canal. **(Ref. 4, p. 299)**

**39. (C)** The primordium of the respiratory system appears at approximately four weeks of development as a diverticulum of the ventral wall of the foregut. The trachea and lungs develop from this diverticulum. **(Ref. 4, pp. 226–235)**

**40. (B)** An absence or insufficient production of surfactant results in a high surface membrane tension that can cause part of the alveolar wall to collapse during expiration. **(Ref. 4, p. 233)**

**41. (E)** Tetralogy of Fallot results from a narrowed right ventricular outflow tract and a large defect of the interventricular septum with the aorta arising superior to the septal defect. This results in a high right ventricular pressure and hypertrophy of the right ventricular myocardium. The aortic valve does not become reduced in size. **(Ref. 4, pp. 331–334)**

**42. (C)** The vitelline duct connects the intestinal loop of the ileum with the yolk sac. If the duct remains patent over its entire length, a direct communication, known as an umbilical fistula, is formed between the umbilicus and intestinal tract. (**Ref. 4,** pp. 277–278)

**43. (B)** The ventral mesentery is prominent at the lower esophagus, stomach, and upper end of the duodenum. The part of the ventral mesentery between the anterior abdominal wall and liver is the falciform ligament. All of the other structures listed are parts of the dorsal mesentery and connect the viscera to the posterior body wall. (**Ref. 4,** pp. 175–176)

**44. (A)** The primitive sex cords are formed from the coelomic epithelium before the primordial germ cells reach the genital ridge. (**Ref. 4,** pp. 281–283)

**45. (B)** Cleft palate is commonly found in trisomy 13-15 but is uncommon in trisomy 21, which is characterized by each of the other conditions listed. (**Ref. 4,** pp. 146–147)

**46. (E)** The tubules of the mesonephros lengthen and form the Bowman's capsule at one end of the tubules. There are successive generations and confluence of the tubules. (**Ref. 4,** p. 267)

**47. (D)** The bladder develops from the caudal ends of the mesonephric ducts and most of the urogenital sinus. Thus, the bladder has both mesodermal and endodermal origins. (**Ref. 4,** pp. 276–277)

**48. (B)** The intermediate mesoderm separates from the paraxial somite mesoderm and forms a lateral cell cluster called the nephrotome. (**Ref. 4,** pp. 267–270)

**49. (C)** The ventral mesentery is a double-walled membrane that extends from the anterior body wall to the lesser curvature of the stomach. Each of the listed structures develops from this membrane except for the mesocolon, which develops from the dorsal mesentery. (**Ref. 4,** p. 243)

**50. (B)** The optic vesicles invaginate and become a double-walled optic cup. The inner layer of the cup is thicker and develops into the neural retina. The outer layer of the cup forms the retinal pigment epithelium. (**Ref. 4,** p. 423)

51. **(A)** During spinal cord devlopment, cellular proliferation and differentiation produce thick lateral walls and the roof and floor plates of the neural canal. The sulcus limitans develops laterally and divides the dorsal or alar plate from the ventral or basal plate. (**Ref. 4,** p. 391)

52. **(C)** The first branchial pouch forms a lateral diverticulum known as the tubotympanic recess, which forms the middle ear cavity. This pouch is lined by endoderm and is a lateral extension of the pharynx. (**Ref. 4,** p. 195)

53. **(C)** When the rectum ends blindly (anorectal agenesis) at the puborectalis muscle, fistulas often develop to the bladder, urethra, or vagina. These defects are the result of incomplete separation of the cloaca by the urorectal septum. (**Ref. 4,** p. 260)

54. **(A)** The derivatives of the foregut extend from the pharynx to the duodenum and include the lower respiratory system, liver, and pancreas. The esophagus, stomach, liver, pancreas, and duodenum are supplied by the celiac artery of the foregut. (**Ref. 4,** p. 257)

55. **(B)** The lateral mesoderm divides into two layers. The outer layer is the somatic mesoderm that lines the outer wall of the intraembryonic coelom and forms the parietal layer of serous membranes. (**Ref. 4,** pp. 265–267)

56. **(C)** The inner layer formed by the splitting of the lateral mesoderm is the splanchnic mesoderm. This splanchnic layer lines the inner wall of the intraembryonic coelom and forms the visceral layer of serous membranes. (**Ref. 4,** p. 43)

57. **(E)** The pleuropericardial membrane is a lateral layer of mesoderm that projects into the thoracic cavity and separates the pericardial and pleural cavities. The phrenic nerve develops in the membrane, which forms the fibrous pericardium in the adult. (**Ref. 4,** pp. 177–178)

**58. (C)** The splanchnic mesoderm is continuous with the wall of the yolk sac until the intraembryonic coelom loses its contact with the extraembryonic coelom. (**Ref. 4,** pp. 43, 56)

**59. (A)** Intraembryonic mesoderm consists of mesodermal cells that invaginate between the epiblast and hypoblast layers in both lateral and cephalic directions. (**Ref. 4,** pp. 53–57)

**60. (B)** The ureteric bud grows into the metanephric tissue and subdivides into twelve or more generations of tubules that give rise to the ureter, renal pelvis, calyces, and collecting tubules. (**Ref. 4,** p. 267)

**61. (C)** The metanephric mesoderm caps the collecting tubules and develops into the proximal and distal convoluted tubules and loop of Henle. (**Ref. 4,** p. 267)

**62. (E)** The mesonephros and gonads are adjacent to each other on either side of the midline, and form an elevation called the urogenital ridge. This ridge is located on each side of the aorta and gives rise to parts of the urinary and genital systems. (**Ref. 4,** p. 265)

**63. (C)** The glomeruli develop from small vesicles and tubules that form within the metanephric mesoderm. The metanephric cap grows over the end of the ureteric bud. (**Ref. 4,** p. 267)

**64. (B)** Bilateral or unilateral absence of the kidney results from an early degeneration of the ureteric bud. The metanephric diverticulum fails to penetrate into the metanephric mesoderm. (**Ref. 4,** p. 274)

**65. (A)** Some rudimentary tubules of the mesonephric duct adjacent to the uterus form the paroophoron in the female. These are located in the broad ligament. (**Ref. 4,** p. 290)

# REFERENCES

1. Carpenter MB: *Core Text of Neuroanatomy,* 4th ed. Baltimore: Williams & Wilkins, 1991.
2. Woodburne RT, Burkel WE: *Essentials of Human Anatomy,* 9th ed. New York: Oxford University Press, 1994.
3. Junqueira LC, Carneiro J, Kelley RO. *Basic Histology,* 7th ed. Norwalk, CT: Appleton & Lange, Inc, 1992.
4. Moore KL, Persaud TVN: *The Developing Human,* 5th ed. Philadelphia: WB Saunders, 1993.